The Student Nurse's Guide to Successful Reflection

Ten Essential Ingredients

The Student Nurse's Guide to Successful Reflection

Ten Essential Ingredients

Second edition

Nicola Clarke

Open University Press

Open University Press
McGraw Hill
Unit 4
Foundation Park
Roxborough Way
Maidenhead
SL6 3UD

Email: emea_uk_ireland@mheducation.com
World wide web: www.mheducation.co.uk

First published 2017
First published in this second edition 2024

Executive Editor: Sam Crowe
Editorial Assistant: Hannah Jones
Content Product Manager: Graham Jones

British Library Cataloguing in Publication Data
A catalogue record of this book is available from the British Library

ISBN-13: 978-0-335-25234-3
ISBN-10: 0-33-525234-6
eISBN: 978-0-335-25235-0

Typeset by Transforma Pvt. Ltd., Chennai, India

Praise Page

Following the success of her first book, this welcome second edition nudges readers to embark on an enlightened journey of reflective practice. This new edition bears all the hallmarks of the original text, with further exploration of reflective practice and cutting-edge content. In this delightful how-to book, the author provides the necessary scaffold for learning, and encourages the reader to reinforce their knowledge through notable exercises and takeaway points. This book is well-organised with clear sections and sub-headings, making it readable and accessible. It is a valuable resource for nursing students, educators and learners from various disciplines. Whether you are a novice learner or seasoned learner, this book provides a unique, engaging, perspective on successful reflection, which is a welcome addition to the arduous academic textbooks on offer.

Shelley O'Connor, Senior Lecturer in Mental Health Nursing, Liverpool John Moores University, UK.

"Although aimed at nursing students, this is an excellent resource for anyone who wants to learn more about themselves and intentionally grow and develop through reflecting on their experience. It offers practical guidance to students on how to engage in reflective practice and critical analysis, but its relevance extends beyond its primary audience. Educators, and in particular personal academic tutors, will find its content invaluable.

Effective personal academic tutoring is pivotal in helping students decipher their educational journey. It empowers them to align their values, interests, and ambitions with their academic pursuits, fostering a path to achieve their aspirations and become their best self. Central to this transformative experience is the practice of reflection and self-examination.

This book gives personal academic tutors an excellent grounding, enabling them to engage their students in the reflective process and to facilitate reflective conversations which empower students to intentionally plan for their future growth and development. Reflecting on their own practice also helps personal academic tutors to understand how and why they support their students in the ways that they do, and how they can do this better.

This book is an engaging and enlightening read. I highly recommend it to all personal tutors, academic advisors and anyone in higher education who guides students to learn more about themselves."

Dr David Grey, UK Advising and
Tutoring Association CEO

"The second edition of this essential book continues to provide practitioners with an accessible and thorough account of reflection's essential ingredients. However, it introduces significant innovations including an emphasis on critical analysis, Socratic questioning and guided reflective conversations. So much more than an academic exercise or professional requirement, reflection is situated as a vital and transformative process through which we can deepen our understanding of self. In convincing and compelling terms, Clarke details how this reflective 'way of being' can not only enable us to become the 'best version of ourselves' but also to become more self-aware, emotionally intelligent and compassionate health care professionals."

Dr Marc Roberts, Visiting Lecturer, Faculty of Health,
Education, and Life Sciences, Birmingham City University, UK

"Reflection is a word frequently used in the nursing world, and from the first day of undergraduate training through to the requirements of NMC revalidation, can create worry and misunderstanding. Reflection and reflective practice, although appearing simple at the outset, can belie the true nature of this incredibly important skill set. What is impressive about Nicola's work is that she has demystified what reflection is, why it is important, and she has really drawn

out the multitude of considerations, skills and understanding that is needed. She has achieved this in a practical, meaningful and 'no nonsense' fashion that really engages the reader. Reflection is far from a 'tick box' exercise, or a way of writing an assignment, Nicola demonstrates that becoming a reflective practitioner, and the skills of this, facilitate the student to explore and gain new depths to their self-awareness, the awareness of others and ultimately, their abilities as a practitioner. This is probably one of the most valuable books a student nurse could use during their training and beyond."

Dr Will Murcott, Senior Lecturer in Mental Health Nursing,
The Open University, UK

Contents

Contents

Foreword

Professional practice in the mid-2020s is complex and becoming more so. Yet to cope with this, there is no rule book to be absorbed and followed (if indeed there ever was). Experienced practitioners and students increasingly need to be alert and able to learn and develop all the time. This would be overwhelming if there were no help at hand. Luckily there is, including in this accessible and informative book by Nicola Clarke.

Nicola helpfully gives ten essential ingredients for reflective practice, to be 'mixed as … for a cake'. The reflective process is an opportunity to stop and spend quality time with ourselves, perhaps meandering and following our flow of feeling or thought. We are inquisitive about everything – what others thought and felt, what happened before and after. We do this to try to make fully rounded sense of experience – both good and bad.

The reflective process develops and even challenges what we think we know about ourselves. It's too easy to take for granted what we think, feel and understand about our world, assuming others see it the same way. It can be hard to realize our whole view of our lives is perspectival, and can differ considerably from others', perhaps those from different backgrounds.

Reflection helps us learn critically from others' understandings which diverge from ours. It also develops an awareness of how our values and belief systems, along with culture, policy and the political sphere, influence who we are in the context of others.

We discover things we need to find out about along the way. Filling these gaps in our knowledge, by reading or talking to knowledgeable colleagues, for example, is fulfilling because it's in response to our own need.

We develop our vast resources for self-understanding, learning how to communicate with our own internal supervisor. This gives confidence, personal knowledge and stability to enquire deeply into our experience. It also strengthens us to be able to enquire into and make sense of our thoughts, feelings and behaviour. It can take courage to face elements of ourselves we might never have faced. Our internal supervisor also supports us in empathic understanding and acceptance of how others perceive us and the experience we had together.

The results of reflective activity might not be obvious. They will, however, be significantly developmental of ourselves as people and professionals. Furthermore, every decision we make as a result of reflection has a 'ripple effect', affecting others as well as ourselves.

The reflective process is personally demanding, Nicola tells us as her final ingredient. We therefore need to be open, honest, willing and courageous to understand better and learn about ourselves. Unconditional positive regard, kindness and compassion towards ourselves will significantly support fruitful reflection.

What does this Guide to Successful Reflection offer? It can help us reframe our attitude to work and study. It can teach us how to step back from busy doing and learn from that doing. This in turn enables us to take responsibility for our actions, and ensure that what we do is in keeping with the values we say we have. A reflective practitioner is one with an open enquiring mind: crucially we can learn this critical way of being. There are no special people who are clever at learning from experience. We focus on what we do, how we do it, when, where and with whom and, significantly, why we act in the ways we do (as well as why others do).

Reflective practice might seem a doddle because it needs little brain-taxing reading and learning, or development of tricky skills. But it makes more intense and subtle demands on us: it requires us to perceive ourselves, as far as we can, from the perspective of others (e.g. the patient); to find out what we urgently need to know or understand; what we know and don't know we know; how we handle our boundaries with others (such as patients and colleagues); what we think, believe and value; and how to ensure our every action is in keeping with those values. We can do all this by writing narratives, stories about our experiences, rereading them, and perhaps rewriting them in specific explorative ways. We learn by becoming authors of our own lives, thus gaining authority over our actions.

Reflective practice is a process with no end. Writing about and reflecting upon a situation, let's say an interaction with a patient, can enable insight into a range of feelings and ideas. Reflection does not end here! Return to it the following week, month, even year, and fresh insight will become apparent.

For this to work for us, rather than be a mere paper exercise, it requires a high level of brave honesty. For it to work really well, however, it also needs a willingness to sit with a friendly co-student over coffee, share reflective writings and have an in-depth talk: an intense, fruitful and rewarding development from everyday sharing of experience.

A doctor once said to me, 'we must stop just doing things, and listen; we must pay attention'. Yes. We must tune the corners of our ears to pick up myriad elements which too often go unnoticed. Later, through writing, we can allow these (which might seem insignificant elements) to come to the forefront of our minds. We can then focus upon their connections and significance. Then, we begin to make sense of our lives creatively and constructively.

Gillie Bolton, PhD
Author of: *Reflective Writing and Professional Development*
5th edition (with Russell Delderfield)

Acknowledgements

First and foremost, I would like to thank again all the students and members of staff who took part in my original research for my educational doctorate. These individuals provided me with the rich data I needed to generate the ideas that underpin the extended description of – and the ten essential ingredients for – successful reflection, which this book is based upon.

I would like to thank my colleagues, students and friends whom I have worked with over the past two decades at Birmingham City University, for providing me with an environment for academic debate and discussion and for listening to me talk at length at times about reflection; for challenging my thinking about reflection when I needed to see other perspectives, acting as my critical friends. My developed thinking, which has resulted in modifications to the extended description, essential ingredients and the additional chapters in this edition, are as a direct result of those conversations.

I would also like to extend a thank you to the students who gave permission for me to use and share some of their writings in this book. That graciousness will help other students to truly understand how to reflect.

I would also like to thank the editorial team at McGraw Hill Education for their support in their diligent editing of my chapters.

I would like to offer a special thank you to Mark Stevens, my mentor and friend, who introduced to me to this world of reflection, and to Mark Hetherington, Marc Roberts and Philip Dee, who have helped me to develop my thinking on reflection, following conversations and many email discussions.

I cannot thank people without giving a special mention to my mum and dad who have always had faith in me, when I may have not, and for supporting me through years and years of study. For being superb role models – as people, as parents and as grandparents. I was one of those individuals who considered themselves *not academic*, but what does this even mean? I have no idea. But what I do know is, with support and a *go for it, open* attitude, we can challenge and shelve those claims we make about ourselves that may really have no meaning and get to where we deserve to be by empowering ourselves to be the *best version of ourselves*!

Finally, I have an amazing daughter who now knows what I do and could now probably teach reflection as well as me!

An introduction to the author

The author of this book Nicola Clarke, EdD, is a Senior Fellow of the Advanced Higher Education Academy and SEDA-recognized doctoral supervisor. Nicola is a registered mental health nurse whose clinical career focused on caring for individuals with a substance misuse issue. Nicola is currently a senior lecturer with over two decades' experience of learning and teaching in a higher education institute, teaching reflection and reflective practice, academic skills and mental health nursing. Nicola is an experienced external examiner and mentor, quality lead for Faculty Recognition of Prior Learning (RPL) and Continuing Professional Development Advisor.

Nicola has published a number of articles in the area of reflection and student assessment, presented at a number of conferences and is the creator of and has published 'Experience, Deconstruction, Implementation: EDI; a new approach to reflective writing for academic purpose' (Clarke, 2021). Nicola is incredibly humbled by the response of students and colleagues to the first edition of this book.

Nicola has one wonderful daughter, three rather lazy cats, has a passion for fitness and lifting weights, and utterly loves Country music.

Beginning our journey into reflection: introducing this wonderful idea of reflection – what it is and why we should do it

Introduction

I have been troubling. In the previous edition of this book, I wrote: 'How many times have you wished you could do things differently? How many times have you wished you could change the way you are, or change the way you think and feel?' (Clarke, 2017: 1); importantly, now, I wish to reframe this. I have read this over and over to myself and each time I walk away with the perception that I am suggesting reflection is only about improvement of self and changing who you are, which is not true. I cannot recount the times I have told my students in class, 'reflection is not about getting better, it is not about improving yourself, it is not about fixing what is wrong, it is about understanding, uncovering the why and making sense of experience. The process of reflection does not wish for you to assume you need to be different or do things differently (you might need to be or do things differently, but this is not the assumption the reflective process makes), the process does not position itself from a negative starting point'. So, having read this, I want you to remember that reflection is about empowerment of self, through understanding of self. Typically, it is not a requirement to need to improve, to be able to reflect. Please know this, you may already be amazing; you just may want to know why you are so amazing so you can continue to be amazing in other facets of your life! This is important to know, this is important to remember, since as a student there will be many occasions when you are told – and are required – to reflect to improve your practice. It is a rare thing to be asked as a student to reflect on when you were amazing, or to reflect on an experience that was incredible for you.

So, let me reframe my thinking and ask, how many times have you wanted to be in more control of your experiences? How often have you wished you knew more about yourself, or knew why you thought and felt the way you did, or responded to particular people or situations in a certain way? Have you ever wanted to know why people respond to you in the manner they do? Have you held onto things, made assumptions, and internalized them as being your responsibility? Have you ever wondered why certain things influence you or give you so much enjoyment, yet others you may dislike or are ambivalent about? Have you ever wished you had a better understanding of why you are, behave, think and feel the way you do? If you have, then continue reading because I am going to introduce you to the wonderful world of reflecting and hopefully engender a curiosity in getting to know yourself.

Developing a curiosity about who you are, what your experiences tell you about yourself, will provide you with information. Information that is

> knowledge specifically about who we are as people, so that we can then use this knowledge to enhance our self-awareness, because self-aware individuals can, should they so wish, also be emotionally intelligent people. The emotionally intelligent person can as a result be an emotionally intelligent healthcare practitioner, educator and, ultimately, the best version of themselves.
>
> (Clarke, 2021: 715)

This is the kind of knowledge about yourself that leads to significant understanding of yourself, that will support transformational change and allow you to adapt, modify and alter behaviours, thoughts and feelings should you choose to do so. Turning this curiosity into reflection and reflective practice is the key to empowering you to become the *best version of you.*

Let us consider another passage from a very familiar character and rather famous bear:

> When you are a Bear of very Little Brain, and you Think of Things, you find sometimes that a Thing which seemed very

Thingish inside of you is quite different when it gets out into the open and has other people looking at it.

(Pooh Bear, in Milne 1928: 78)

This is Pooh Bear discussing an incident with Piglet where he felt terribly guilty having had the great idea of throwing stones into the water to 'hoosh' Eeyore (who was currently floating down river having been bounced into it by Tigger) to safety on the opposite side of the river. Having picked up a very large stone, Pooh threw it into the river with the intention of missing Eeyore. As the large stone hit the water, however, Eeyore sank but emerged on the other side and to the safety of the riverbank. Pooh is told by Eeyore that the stone was dropped on him, which left Pooh feeling terrible and having feelings of guilt. However, Piglet, who observed the whole experience, enlightened Pooh and told him he had not dropped the stone on Eeyore, which made Pooh feel considerably better. I hope that as you continue reading this book, in particular Chapter 9, you will realize the value of feedback in the generation of information about who you are.

I would like to welcome you to this second edition of the *Student Nurse's Guide to Successful Reflection*. I have been utterly astounded by the reception to the first edition, so much so in fact, that I wanted to create a second edition to incorporate new chapters, to give you, the reader, some new information that I truly hope will enhance and extend the knowledge you may have gained about reflection from that first book. Since writing the first edition, my colleagues of similar thinking and I have been working hard to continue to ignite a passion for reflection and reflective practice in our students across the health, education and life science courses. Listening to you, the students, and taking on board your responses and the responses of my peers to the first edition is what generated the thinking that there should be a second edition.

As a result, the introduction to this edition has been rewritten as I really would like us to fully establish and progress our understanding of reflection and the reflective process. Importantly, I want us to explore the purposeful use of the word 'experience' as a replacement for 'event', 'action' or 'incident' when referring to reflection-on/reflection-in/reflection-before. I am going to advocate for the importance of telling your narrative or story, how telling your narrative is self-care and quite possibly one of the most important aspects of the reflective process. The aim of this book remains the same – to support you in developing the necessary skills and attitude for successful reflection. And, more importantly, engender a 'way of being' that naturalizes the reflective process for you and hopefully instils a sense of passion towards reflective practice – with the aim of fostering a level of emotional intelligence. An emotional intelligence that allows you as practitioners to be able to use yourselves intelligently and therapeutically within the helping, caring and educating relationship.

Several of the chapters in this book are centred on an approach to reflection and reflective practice that emerged from the findings of a person-centred enquiry into the teaching and learning of reflection and reflective practice (Clarke, 2014). The research findings produced *ten essential ingredients for successful reflection* (see Figure 1.1) and an extended description of reflection.

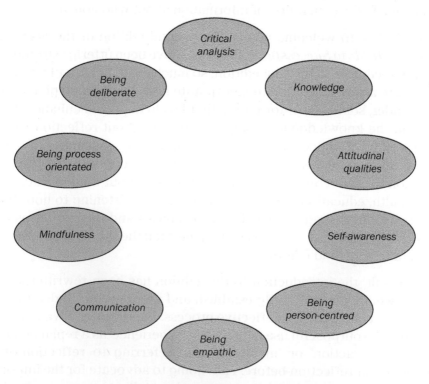

Figure 1.1 The ten essential ingredients for successful reflection
Source: Clarke (2017: 2).

Although some of the content and language in the extended description and detailing of each ingredient (you will notice I have changed the title of the first ingredient from *academic skills* to *critical analysis* and the tenth ingredient from *being strategic* to *being deliberate*) has altered to account for my own developing thinking and knowledge about reflection, with some updates in relation to examples provided, the essence of the message conveyed in these chapters has not changed from the first edition.

Figure 1.1 lays out for you ten key ingredients for reflection that will be explored in pairs in Chapters 2–6. These ten ingredients combined (mixed as you would combine the ingredients for a cake) can be used independently as an approach to the way you reflect, or should you feel you need that extra structure, in combination with a reflective model or cycle that will provide you with a framework within which to reflect in whatever mode you choose. Later chapters are dedicated to exploring how the process of reflection itself can in fact become a framework for reflection that empowers use of the ten essential ingredients in a non-prescriptive way, how to write reflectively using a very specific framework of Experience-Deconstruction-Implementation (EDI) (Clarke, 2021) and, finally, how to engage in reflection through facilitated reflective conversation.

Schön and the swampy lowlands

Before any of us can engage in reflection or reflective practice, or facilitate reflection in another person, it is of absolute importance that we have a good theoretical understanding of what this term means. Without a full understanding of this term, the many reflective models and frameworks there are to support movement through the reflective process will be used incorrectly. So, having the right understanding means we are practising reflection without an assumed knowledge base. Roberts (2015) and Thompson and Thompson (2023) believe that the popularization of some terms (buzz words) and extensive use of good ideas leads to oversimplification of those terms and ideas, and assumptions that those using them understand them. Unfortunately, it is my experience that reflection and reflective practice have fallen prey to this. As a result, reflection is used at times superficially without doing justice to its complex nature (Thompson and Thompson, 2023), and is 'tagged on to a variety of activities in an attempt to add credibility to them' (Roberts, 2015: 21).

Furthermore, reflection has been, and is often still, promoted and taught as evaluation of practice: what went well, what didn't go well and what will you do to enhance practice? But in the health, education and life sciences professions, we know that clinical practice is far more complex than this and can involve uncertainty, troubling, value conflict, uniqueness, interpersonal connectedness and intuition – referred to by Schön as 'the swampy lowlands' (1983: 43).

Schön, who was one of the strongest advocates of reflection (Thompson and Thompson, 2023), used the analogy of the swampy lowlands as a way of creating value beyond that of technical rationality, with Schön describing technical rationality as 'instrumental problem solving made rigorous by the application of scientific theory and technique' (1983: 21). Today you may hear this referred to as evidence-based practice. So, when we address what went well and did not go so well and create an action plan for improvement, I would suggest we are not in Schön's swampy lowlands where the messes and intricacies of people are, but we are in the high, hard ground of technical rationality where we are evaluating the mechanics of practice.

> In the varied topography of professional practice, there is a high, hard ground where practitioners can make effective use of research-based theory and technique, and there is a swampy lowland where situations are confusing 'messes' incapable of technical solution. The difficulty is that the problems of the high ground, however great their technical interest, are often relatively unimportant to clients or to the larger society, while in the swamp are the problems of greatest human concern.
>
> (Schön, 1983: 42)

I am by no means suggesting that evaluating our practice is not an absolute *must*. But in remaining on the high ground of technical rationality, Schön (1983) cautions us that, as practitioners, we can become incredibly proficient at *knowing in* action. Where our technical knowledge is highly *known* to us, we become so good and almost inherently robotic in following the evidence base or protocol that we miss opportunities 'to think about what we are doing' (Schön, 1983: 61). Schön advised that if this happens, there is a potential for us to become 'inattentive to the phenomena that do not fit the categories of knowing in action' (ibid.). Then we are at risk of attempting to force experiences to fit the mould of our technical rationality. Let me give you an example.

When I was working as a clinician, my case load was predominantly of people who were injecting heroin daily. At that time, there were less than a handful of consultant psychiatrists across the country whose specialism was addiction. As a result, I made it my mission to *know* the evidence base on addiction as much as I could and to have as many skills as possible. I became very proficient as a practitioner and my *knowing in action* became second nature. But the people I cared for are human beings. Human beings come with thoughts, feelings, perceptions, history, values and beliefs, and all these unique people came with significantly distinctive experiences of doing the same thing – using heroin. If I had only employed technical rationality to evaluate my practice, never exploring the interpersonal connections I had with the people I worked with, never exploring how they affected me, how I affected them – maybe controversially, I would boldly say, I would only have ever been mediocre at my job!

I now work as an educator in a university setting. I teach an introduction to reflection on average once a month to different students on different courses across the health, education and life sciences. The technicalities of my lesson are more or less the same, the information I want to convey is the same, my Power-Point presentation the same. However, how I use myself to convey the information, to engage my students, to motivate them to want to listen to me, to become interested in reflection is always different. I am the vessel that my lesson is conveyed through. After twenty years of teaching and reflecting on my lessons with students from different programmes, I am becoming more masterful in using the vessel, which is me, to convey the lesson. I have a much greater understanding of how different students respond to me, and I to them. I have adapted and modified my behaviours when I perceive a class is not responding to my style productively. I have reflected on these adaptations and analysed student responses to me. I am always learning about the context of me and the interpersonal connections I have in my teaching environments. This helps me to be the *best version of myself*; this helps me to ensure my lessons are received well.

'I/you/we are the vessel through which the professional practice radiates. Moving beyond technical rationality and engaging in reflection, by delving into and exploring the messiness of the swampy lowlands – lowlands that contain the humanness of values, beliefs, feelings, interpersonal connections and the influence of culture, policy and politics – will allow you to be the master of your own vessel. The vessel which is the vehicle through which our practice emanates. Understanding your vehicle, learning to drive the vehicle of self with knowledge and authority, is what will enable you to be an amazing practitioner/professional.'

My hope, therefore, is that you will be able to determine that just evaluating practice experience, or just engaging in technical rationality, is not reflection or reflective practice.

When we explore what reflection is here, we do so by situating it within the health, education and life science professions. The writers that we explore here would possibly position themselves within these fields and although this book includes in its title the words 'student nurse's guide', what we discuss here will support all professionals in the health, education and life sciences. So let us explore what we understand the notion of reflection to mean.

Exploring the meaning of reflection

Whether you are new to reflection or have read the first edition of this book and are already an effective reflective practitioner, have a go at the following exercise, where I ask you to define reflection but also explore what experiences have given you your knowledge. I am hoping that by the end of this book, you will understand that where you get your knowledge from is as important as having the knowledge, and that it is our experiences that provide and generate knowledge.

Exercise 1.1: Characterizing reflection

- Have a go at writing your own definition of reflection and then compare it with those that follow.
- Then ask yourself: *What experiences have I had that have given me the knowledge to write this definition?*

In considering reflection for educators, Robins et al. (2003) suggested that reflection and reflective practice are processes that support and enable deep understanding of self and personal philosophy in relation to the changing environment of their classrooms, with both White (2004) and Wieringa (2011) recognizing reflection as a form of purposeful thinking that generates self-knowledge and understanding. Here it is suggested we are using reflection as a way of developing knowledge of self in the context of others, those others being: those we care for, those who care for those we care for, and those we educate and those we work alongside. Bolton and Delderfield (2018), who have specialist interest in reflection and have written extensively, state that reflection is an in-depth consideration of our experiences where we focus on our thoughts and feelings about what occurred and what we perceived we were part of. These authors emphasize exploring the *why* of the experience, using theory to help generate information about the *why*, or as I tell my students – we use the theory to bring objectivity into the subjective. Using all the wonderful literature that is out there can provide us with knowledge we do not yet have, can offer us different perspectives on how we can view our experiences, can confirm our thinking and can help challenge our assumptions. Don't be afraid to read when reflecting but as I tell my students, read *deeply, not just widely*.

In a nursing context, Melanie Jasper, a highly respected nurse, editor and prolific writer on reflection, who I was fortunate enough to meet when she acted as one of my viva examiners for my educational doctorate (and boy did she make me prove my worth!), wanted us to know that

> ... reflective practice means we learn by thinking about things that have happened to us and looking at them in a different way, which enables us to take action. Reflective practice can be summarised as having three components.
>
> 1   Things (experiences) happen to a person
> 2   The reflective processes that enable the person to learn from those experiences
> 3   The action that results from the new perspectives that are taken.
>
> (2013: 4)

As we can see, Jasper (2013) summarizes reflective practice as Experience- Reflection-Action (ERA). She advises all three elements need to be present for reflective practice to occur. So when discussing reflective practice here, what we mean is using the knowledge we have gained from reflection on or before a previous experience to inform our future experience. Also, when we are reflecting during the experience or 'in-action' as Schön (1983) described, we are exploring self in the moment, and using that knowledge to adapt behaviours, thoughts and feelings as we experience them to inform what is occurring at the time. Roberts further advised us that 'engaging in the reflective process would mean a rigorous questioning and challenging of those factors that craft thoughts and feelings and drive behaviour, with a view to developing alternative ways of thinking, feeling and acting in future situations' (2015: 21). And Clarke (2021, 2022) more recently wants us to know that reflection is the immersion in and analysis of experiences, exploring who we are as a person within the context of others and the wider political sphere, with the purpose of generating knowledge about what constitutes 'I'.

Here we have acknowledged just a few authors who have written about reflection across the professional disciplines, and as I have always advised my students when reviewing the literature on reflection, to one degree or another the essence of what is being articulated in the wonderful world of information about reflection is the same. We can see here the similarity between the disciplines of education and health. We can maybe acknowledge that not at any point do these authors refer to reflection as simply an evaluation of practice with no reference to exploration of self. All these authors note that reflection and reflective practice are about you and your experiences. So, maybe we can conclude that reflection is exploring the movie of your life, using a critical and analytical process to understand your experiences so you can uncover the essence of their meanings. We then draw upon the knowledge gained to formulate conclusions about our experiences and what constitutes 'I'. Importantly, we use this knowledge to move forward with either confirmation and/or validation of our sense of self, to inform experiences we are in the moment of, or to inform future experiences. But what we must do in reflective practice, is use this knowledge to elevate our understanding of self in the context of others – this is what can enhance practice. This supports emotional intelligence, and who wouldn't want to be an emotionally intelligent person and professional?

Look now at the explanation of reflection you provided in Exercise 1.1. Review this taking into consideration what we have just discussed. Is your explanation of reflection like any of those we have discussed, or are there differences? You may, perhaps, find your explanation is more akin to evaluation of practice where we consider how things went. You may realize that the missing aspect is the added dimension of the self. As we now know, reflecting is so much more than just evaluating the mechanics of an event or incident. An important take-away is that you will notice that not one of the authors we discussed talks about *being better* or *improving*. Reflection does not assume you need to be better, or do better, or fix what went wrong. *The process of reflection assumes a neutral value position, a position that assumes you wish to understand, you wish to generate meaning.*

I suggested early on in this chapter that this edition of the book centres around the ten essential ingredients for successful reflection to occur, which aligns with an extended description of reflection – this has not changed from the first edition. However, I have modified my original extended description to take into consideration my own developed and altered thinking about reflection. The resulting revised version of the extended description of reflection is given in Box 1.1.

Box 1.1: A revised extended description of reflection

Reflection is an essential, engaging process that allows the reflector to frame and reframe their reality that is, and has been experienced moment by moment. Actively participating in the reflective process – that is, in, on or before an experience – requires us to tell our story and meander through that narrative, allowing ourselves to move where our thoughts and feelings wish to take us. It requires us to utilize skills of communication, to communicate with ourselves authentically, to become our own person-centred enquirer, understanding ourselves in relation to experiences we are about to have, are having or have had, empathically and with accuracy. Then stepping beyond the self and using this knowledge gained to understand how we may then have influenced those around us. To be fully immersed in this process, we must be open to learning about what constitutes 'I', leaving arrogance and complacency at the door, be kind and compassionate enough to offer ourselves unconditional positive regard, be actively engaged in mindfulness, and consciously aware of the self in our moments.

Through a critical, analytical lens, we need to explore our experiences within the frame of how our history/background and current locus, culture and context influence who we are in our moments. Reflection requires us to open ourselves up to sourcing and learning new knowledge if the knowledge is not already known to us. And using that new knowledge gained to fill gaps in our current knowledge, challenge our preconceived notions and assumptions, and offer alternative ways of viewing experience to generate sense-making, thus creating information that can lead to personal and professional development. When we are fully open to and engaged in the process, reflection has the potential to empower us to be the best version of ourselves and inform our future experiences.

On reading this book, having worked your way through all the chapters, you will have a thorough understanding of what reflection is, how the ten essential ingredients support understanding of the extended description, and how they enable you to embody the reflective process.

The word experience and showcasing the reflective process

You may have noticed I tend to use the word experience when referring to what we are reflecting on. I am very mindful of not using the words incident, action or event. Have a go at the following exercise and see if you can draw conclusions as to why I prefer the word experience(s).

Exercise 1.2: Understanding use of the word 'experience'

Jot down your thoughts to the following questions:

- If I asked you to reflect on a critical incident, what type of incident would you choose?
- When you have previously been asked to reflect on a critical incident, what type of incident did you choose to reflect on?
- If I asked you to reflect on an event, what type of experience would you constitute as an event?
- If I asked you to reflect on action, what type of action would you choose?

When I ask my students to reflect on a critical *incident*, they almost always choose something significant that was also negative for them. The term critical incident for them does not conjure up anything positive. My nursing students are consistently advised to recall experiences that were significant for them, where the word significance is usually framed as something non-positive. I am aware that in NHS trusts, staff are encouraged to reflect on 'never events', which again are usually negative. I don't think there is a trust policy that says you must reflect on something that you have done well or has made you happy, or that you were ambivalent about! And debriefing sessions, when facilitated well, can assist reflection, but again debriefs often emerge because of a critical incident and are influenced by experiences of a negative nature. This can create a difficult and non-positive relationship with reflection, where we are conditioned to perceive reflection as a tool to use when we and our practice need fixing and improving. Reflecting can therefore become onerous, anxiety-provoking and challenging in a non-productive way.

Let's now consider the word *event* – to me, this word implies something big. Events to me are concerts, fun runs or other occasions large in the eyes of others. If we use the word event, then we are teaching ourselves that our experiences need to be large, perceived as significant by others to warrant reflecting on. We may be conditioning ourselves to understand that reflection is only worth undertaking when something huge has occurred. This stops us from recognizing the learning that can also come from those tiny moments in life, from the brief encounters we have, from the flutter of emotions that come and go, and from the thoughts that pop in and out of our heads.

Returning to Schön (1983), he thought that reflection requires us to delve into the swampy lowlands of humanness, so using the terms reflection *on-* and *in-action* could be suggested to be at odds with the notion of the swampy lowlands. Using the word *action* reduces reflection to a review of something practical – a lesson delivered, an injection given, an assessment undertaken. A review of the mechanics of practice. So, I think using the word action, as with the words incident and event, does reflection a disservice and does not reveal meaningfully the true sense of reflection.

This is why I prefer the word experience. Reflection on/in/before experience. Experience means a *happening*, and every moment we have lived, or are living, or are going to live is a happening. The word experience allows us to recognize that every moment we have in life can be perceived as something to reflect on. These moments do not need to be perceived as an incident, or large enough to warrant being called an event, or a particular action we have taken. These moments can be anything that have encouraged us to think, feel and behave. We may not even class these moments as significant, but that doesn't mean we cannot learn from them.

When we were allowed to emerge from lockdown during the Covid-19 pandemic, when the coffee shops opened and we could drink our cup of coffee sitting outside, what a moment that was for me. An experience that generated thoughts and feelings within me that I connected with. I was sitting drinking my favourite Caffè Nero flat white on a chair and my view was … a large concrete car park! But I could see people, I could hear people, I could observe and watch, I could smell my fresh coffee, I could feel the sun and wind, I felt peace, calm, safety. The feelings I had resonated so much with me that I choose to reflect on this experience. This non-event, non-critical incident taught me things I did not know about myself. Reflecting on coffee drinking in that moment helped me to make sense of why I love coffee shops so much, why I people watch, why I get enjoyment from it, and it helped me to uncover the *why* of what the notion of loneliness and what being alone meant for me. Not bad from just drinking coffee.

I invite you to have a go at the following exercise. Give yourself permission to enjoy it.

Exercise 1.3: Your non-critical incident, non-event moments

Jot down your memory of an experience that resonated with you, using the prompts:

Give yourself permission for this to be anything from your personal or professional life.
Give yourself permission for this not to be an event or critical incident.
Give yourself permission to choose any moment in your life.

- Where were you?
- What were you doing?
- What thoughts did you have?
- What feelings did you have?
- How did you behave?
- What do you think of how others behaved?
- What could you smell?
- What could you see?
- What thoughts did it leave you with afterwards?
- How did you feel afterwards?

Now that we have a good understanding of what reflection is, let us review its purpose and consider the importance of reflection.

Importance and purpose?

Before we get into detail about the purpose and importance of reflection, have a go at the following exercise. Hopefully, you will have begun to add to the knowledge you already have about reflection based on what you have read so far.

Exercise 1.4: Purpose and importance

Jot down your thoughts on the following questions:

- What is the purpose of reflection?
- Why is reflection important?

Any student undertaking a health, education or life sciences course will be made aware that at some point they will be required by their professional governing body to reflect as part of revalidation processes and to ensure they meet standards of proficiency. The Nursing and Midwifery Council (NMC) requires nurses to have a reflective dialogue with another NMC registrant every three years. During this discussion, the registrant must reflect on experiences of continuing professional development (CPD) that align to the NMC Code of

Professional Conduct (2018b). As part of their Standards of Proficiency (2023), the Health & Care Professions Council (HCPC) requires all members to know the value of reflection and to be able to reflect; the HCPC also promotes reflection as a way of recording and documenting CPD. In a joint statement by the nine health and care professions regulators, ensuring reflection is not perceived as simply a tick-box exercise and that employers and employees devote time and effort to reflect are considered to be of paramount importance (NMC, 2019). According to Agnew (2022), these nine health and care professions regulators perceive the purposes of reflection to be helping staff to make sense of situations, putting learning into action, sharing knowledge, and enhancing the safety of care and education. So, we can see here that the purpose of reflection becomes a way of supporting our ability to meet standards of proficiency, revalidate and enhance practice.

But let us move beyond these professional requirements, which might have us view reflection as a bureaucratic exercise. Boyd and Fales wrote that reflection 'is the core difference between whether a person repeats the same experience several times becoming highly proficient at one behaviour, or learns from experience in such a way that he or she is cognitively or affectively changed' (1983: 100). This is important because within the health, education and life science professions, the environment is forever changing and this change is influenced by many factors, including the human factor. We don't want to be stuck with only one behaviour; we want to be able to adapt, make sense of ourselves, alter our course of direction if it is no longer working for us.

You have all most likely heard of Graham Gibbs. He advised:

> It is not sufficient simply to have an experience in order to learn. Without reflecting upon this experience, it may quickly be forgotten, or its learning potential lost. It is from the feelings and thoughts emerging from this reflection that generalisations or concepts can be generated. And it is generalisations that allow new situations to be tackled effectively.
>
> (1998: 9)

Clarke told us that:

> The principal purpose of reflection through discourse, mindfulness, or writing is the generation of information that equates to

knowledge. Knowledge specifically about who we are as people, so that we can then use this knowledge to enhance our self-awareness, because self-aware individuals can, should they so wish, also be emotionally intelligent people. The emotionally intelligent person can as a result be an emotionally intelligent healthcare practitioner, educator and, ultimately, the best version of themselves.

(2021: 714)

Maybe we can determine here that these authors are highlighting the significance of the learning potential of experience, that engaging in the reflective process purposefully moves us to explore and analyse experiences so that learning about self can occur. We can assert that the purpose of reflection is to generate information, and this information can be used to inform future experiences. Have a look at Figure 1.2 to view the fundamental purpose of reflection.

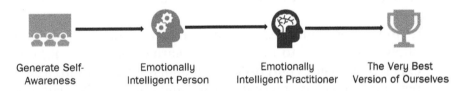

| Generate Self-
Awareness | Emotionally
Intelligent Person | Emotionally
Intelligent Practitioner | The Very Best
Version of Ourselves |

Figure 1.2 The fundamental purpose of reflection

But why is it so important to reflect? We already know from our professional governing bodies that there is a perception that reflection can enhance practice. I would agree that it can, if undertaken correctly. If you open yourself up to getting to know yourself and draw upon the wider sphere of knowledge drawn from feedback from others in your experience, literature, policy, culture and context, you can not only make sense of yourself but fill gaps in your knowledge, challenge your preconceived ideas and ways of practising, and allow different perspectives of your experience to be considered – all of this will enhance practice. But there are also other important reasons. Ghaye suggested that reflection allows the healthcare professional to seek their own voice, 'an authentic voice and one that enables them to talk about their experiences and their ability, or not, to learn from the work that they do' (2000: 59).

I want to focus here on the *authentic voice*. Advocating for yourself to not only have a voice, but to hear your own voice, is very important and the reflective process – as hopefully you will see when you read the other chapters in this book – can give you a place to find this authenticity, this realness. This is not easy to do and requires you to have certain attitudinal qualities as a reflector, which are detailed later in the book.

Taking the time to reflect and provide the climate for authenticity to occur, we could also view as self-care. Giving yourself permission to explore your experiences, offering yourself the unconditional positive regard to create a climate where honesty comes to the fore, might for the first time allow you to truly give yourself permission to acknowledge your accurate thoughts and feelings about your lived experiences. There have been times when I have told myself off for having certain thoughts or wished I hadn't felt a certain way and have tried to push these feelings away, taking time out to recognize me and hear me is validating. Elsewhere, I have highlighted the importance of the self-care factor in reflection:

> … [reflection] validates our narrative empathically; a notion often only applied to those we are caring for. Analysing our experience ensures purposeful thinking, not rumination, which potentially resolves internal conflict and remedies distortion of experience, leading to irrational guilt.
>
> (Clarke, 2022: 17)

Reflection therefore is multipurpose, and first and foremost it creates a climate for the understanding and growth of self or 'I'.

The reflective process

We now know what reflection is, we know what its purpose is, and we know why it is important. Before moving on to the next chapter, we must capture what the process of reflection is. I imagine you have been introduced to many reflective frameworks, models and cycles that can support your movement through the reflective process, but my experience is such that we don't tend to teach our students what the actual process of reflection is – and reflection is a process, a process that is not governed by rigid criteria, strict rules or formulas. The reflective process has elements that are dipped into and out of, that overlap and elements that cannot occur without each other and without you at the centre.

Have a go at the following exercise, and become a creator of information.

Exercise 1.5: The reflective process

Try designing your own reflective process based upon what you know about reflection so far.

Taking into account and blending everything we have learned so far, we can see that one element of the reflective process is immersion within our experiences. Whether we are recalling an experience to reflect on the past in order to draw conclusions to either validate knowledge of self or to inform future experiences; or we are being acutely mindfully present within an experience as it is occurring in order to be able to inform the experience as it is occurring; or whether we are considering the potentiality of an experience before it occurs in order to have more information about ourselves prior to the experience – all three require immersion in an experience.

The element of immersion within our experiences is where we become our own storyteller. Where we subjectively and non-critically tell the movie of our lived experience. Where we give ourselves permission to own thoughts and feelings. Narratives, or stories of our lived experience, can bring to life our 'daily theories-in-use, or the values-in use which underpin them' (Bolton and Delderfield, 2018: 79), theories and values that we often have little conscious knowledge of and are often not aware of, as these are built on implicitly known or tacit knowledge (Bolton and Delderfield, 2018). Knowledge that we have accumulated through past experiences, but we are not consciously aware how it influences us. Somewhat controversially, I would suggest that this element of immersion in our experiences in order to bring to life these daily theories in use, becomes the most important aspect of the reflective process. This is the element that allows us to connect with ourselves, validates our stories or narrative. This is the element that empowers an authentic voice in us. This is the element that allows for the critical lens to be used through which to then view the lived experience and for the analytical exploration to occur. Without immersion within our experiences, what do we have to analyse and explore and learn from?

We have discussed the need to view our experiences through a critical lens, to critically analyse the experiences we have. It is this critical analysis that generates knowledge, meaning and sense-making. This critical analysis helps us to uncover the *why* of an experience. Without this we cannot draw conclusions. Now remember, criticality is not the same as critique or just addressing what was good or bad. Criticality is exploration and investigation and is discussed in depth in later chapters. It is this critical lens that will generate knowledge about who we are that will allow us to draw conclusions. So, a further element of the reflective process is to draw conclusions about what the analysis means before moving onto the final element, considering what to do with this new knowledge. Importantly, when considering what to do with this new knowledge you have of yourself, give yourself permission, if you so wish, to simply be okay with what you already know. It does not always mean an action plan needs to be created. So, let's look at the reflective process.

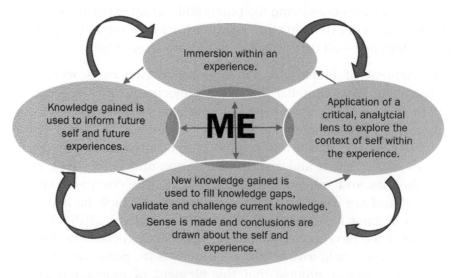

Figure 1.3 The reflective process

Figure 1.3 shows how the elements of the process overlap, with you/ me/I at the centre. This overlapping gives us permission to move fluidly through the four elements in an interconnected way. The process allows us to *dip in and out* of each element, moving backwards, forwards or sideways as determined by the organic nature of reflection. Existing reflective models/frameworks/cycles, some of which were discussed in the first edition, will support movement through this process. Some in a very structured, mechanical way. And some will be more helpful to you than others. Most importantly, you must understand that reflection is a process with four interconnected core elements. Chapter 7 will detail how the reflective process itself can become a framework to empower you to move through the reflective process.

The next five chapters will guide you through the ingredients required for successful reflection to occur and demonstrate to you how each ingredient is used during the reflective process and how each aligns with the extended description of reflection.

Key points that can be taken from this chapter are:

- Reflection is a process with four interconnected elements.
- Reflection is a critical and analytical exploration of experience that focuses on the self in the context of others and the wider sphere of culture and context.
- Reflection is about making sense of experiences to enable the *why* to be uncovered.
- Reflection recognizes the human element of experiences and its influence on how we behave within those experiences.
- Reflection can enhance practice as it can enable the development of emotional intelligence.
- Reflection can explore any experience we have in life, from the minutia of moments to the significant experiences in our professions.
- Adapting our behaviours during an experience, or using the knowledge gained from reflection on experience to inform future experiences, becomes reflective practice.
- Reflection is a form of self-care.
- Reflection allows for authentic storytelling and a challenging of the narrative we create, bringing objectivity into the subjective.
- Reflection supports us to explore the influence and impact we have on those around us.
- Reflection helps us to become critically analytical thinkers, able to truly explore experiences and as a result choose to change practice and personal behaviours.

Critical analysis and knowledge

2

Essential ingredient #1: Critical analysis

Reflecting does not stop at the experience, but continues with an exploration of the experience prior to, during or after, through a critical, analytical lens. This critical analysis is inquisitive in nature, embodying curiosity and generated by the need to make sense of the experience and the quest for knowledge, particularly knowledge that can bridge the theory–practice gap and so be meaningful to the practice or personal experience. New knowledge gained is then amalgamated with the old and current knowledge, from which the person can then synthesize a new way of being leading to transformational change or expand and develop the current way of being.

Essential ingredient #2: Knowledge

The individual, in order to analyse, and reflect upon what they are experiencing in the clinical or personal setting, needs to have a level of knowledge that they can refer to and position their experience within. This knowledge enables objectivity to be brought into the subjective, filling knowledge gaps and challenging perception. If they do not have the existing knowledge, they need to know how to source the knowledge so that they may bridge that theory–practice gap and enhance their ability to understand the experience they are reflecting on.

Learning outcomes

By the end of this chapter, you will be able to:

- Recognise the difference between the descriptive storytelling aspect of the reflective process and reflection that is analytical in nature and therefore moving through the reflective process.
- Use the skills of critical analysis to explore your experiences to generate sense-making.
- Identify the importance of knowledge recall and knowledge sourcing and apply this when reflecting.
- Know how powerful the gaining of knowledge can be and how it can support transformational change.

Now that we have a solid understanding of reflection and know what the process of reflection is, the aim of this chapter is to explore the difference between remaining in the very important storytelling, narrative aspect of the reflective process and moving into the analytical, sense-making aspect of it. We will be identifying the roles that knowledge and the skills of critique and analysis play in supporting the application of the analytical lens through which we will need to explore our experiences. These skills are essential not only for the reflective process but essential also in the caring and educating professions. Nurses, healthcare practitioners and educators not only need to be compassionate, caring and kind but also need to be able to work within an informed evidence-based framework, possessing the cognitive skills of decision-making and problem-solving (Wilkinson, 1996). Being able to source and critically review literature, research and clinical guidelines can support safe and effective practice (Atkins, 2004; Taylor, 2006).

Let us now take a look at our first essential ingredient – *critical analysis*.

Critical analysis

Essential ingredient #1: Critical analysis

Reflecting does not stop at the experience, but continues with an exploration of the experience prior to, during or after, through a critical, analytical lens. This critical analysis is inquisitive in nature, embodying curiosity and generated by the need to make sense of the experience and the quest for knowledge, particularly knowledge that can bridge the theory–practice gap and so be meaningful to the practice or personal experience. New knowledge gained is then amalgamated with the old and current knowledge, from which the person can then synthesize a new way of being leading to transformational change or expand and develop the current way of being.

First of all, for those of you who have read the first edition of this book, you will notice the name of ingredient #1 has changed. Again, from my own developing thinking and considering the message I wanted to convey to you, I have changed it from academic skills to critical analysis. Critical thinking – and as a result critical analysis – is, in my humble opinion, a very important skill to have. It is a skill that is not only required in academia but is transferable to every facet of life. It is also important for successful reflection, so the change in name helps facilitate this.

Critical analysis, critical thinking, being critically analytical and viewing things through a critical lens will be used interchangeably here, as it is my experience they often are used this way and to be honest I am not sure there is any real difference between them. My more esteemed colleagues, however, might have a different opinion. But what I do know is that critical analysis, being critically analytical, is amazing and opens us up to a whole world of possibilities and potential alternatives, teaches us to question, to explore and to interrogate, and to not take anything at face value. It quite literally is wonderful. When I teach critical analysis as part of teaching academic skills to undergraduate and postgraduate nurses, seasoned healthcare practitioners and educators, I always ask them about previous experiences of academic writing or presenting. Their responses are often:

'My feedback tells me I am too descriptive.'

'Apparently I need to be more analytical.'

'I have been told to explore more.'

'I don't know how to be analytical.'

Being critically analytical is the vehicle that allows us to explore that most important part of the reflective process: our story, our narrative. Being critically analytical enables us to meander through our story. It enables us to ask probing questions, to explore how the different elements of our story connect, break off to form smaller stories and then reconnect to allow us to make sense of the whole story.

It is empowered by curiosity. If you are curious, you will ask questions, you will want to investigate, you will want to interrogate, you will want to know, you will be interested in you and the meaning of you. If you are curious, you will never take things at face value and you will pause to consider whether something is sensible or justified or the argument presented is persuasive (Chatfield, 2018).

Have a go at the following exercise.

Exercise 2.1: Defining critical analysis

Jot down what you think critical analysis is. How would you describe it to me? What can you remember from the teaching you have had on critical thinking?

So, what is critical analysis?

To be critically analytical, we must first understand what it means to think in a critical manner. Critical thinkers in nursing have been described as truth-seekers, demonstrating open-mindedness, suspending judgement, having an intellectual curiosity that allows them to seek answers to questions about themselves and their practice (Paul, 1993). Nurses – and anyone else for that matter who practice critical thinking – avoid making assumptions. In fact, historically, critical thinking has been described as reflective thinking. Dewey described critical thinking as 'the active, persistent and careful consideration of a belief … in the light of the grounds which support it' (1910: 6), while Ennis advised us that it is 'reasonable reflective thinking focused on deciding what to believe or do' (1996: 166). Hanscomb (2017) wanted us to recognize *us* in the critical thinking process – that when we are arguing a case, listening to our peers or colleagues, and determining if their argument is persuasive or has merit, what we argue and what we determine can be susceptible to our own moods, emotions, personality, culture and context. That this can cloud our judgement if we are not aware of self within our critical thinking.

Egege described critical thinking as follows: it 'is the process of analysing, evaluating and critiquing information in order to increase our understanding and knowledge of reality' (2020: 3). Egege suggested that as a result of this critical process, which utilizes such skills as assessment, evaluation and reasoning, we can generate valid conclusions that are persuasive in nature due to the objectivity demonstrated in the creation of the argument.

Any student or nurse who thinks critically about what they have experienced, or are experiencing, sees beyond the surface of what is occurring and seeks answers in an attempt to understand what is really occurring. To think critically, we need to gather information, accumulate and evaluate the evidence, understand our own assumptions and beliefs about the experience and what has informed them, draw on current knowledge, recognize and fill the gaps in our knowledge, from which we synthesize the information and ultimately draw conclusions. A critical thinker doesn't just see the trees; they get lost in the wood and will question each turn and review each path and its implications before emerging on the other side.

During the critical thinking process, the student or nurse will analyse the information that their intellectual curiosity is bringing to their conscious mind. To be critical of the information, they will acknowledge the material and break it down into its constituent parts, before determining how the parts are related to each other, influence each other and the implications of this for an overall structure.

When I ask my students what critical analysis is in the reflective process, it is common for them to say:

'I should be just looking back at my practice and identifying what went well and did not go well.'

'I don't know how to be analytical when reflecting; isn't it just stating one person's argument and finding the opposite. I don't know how I do this when it's just my thoughts.'

'Why do I need to use literature and analysis when I am writing about myself?'

To help my students to understand what critical analysis is, therefore, I ask them to reflect on their roles at work in the clinical area, or on life in general in relation to the decisions they make. I ask them to consider the decision-making process and I ask them to take me step by step through what they would do to make a fully informed choice. What I highlight during the discussion is where critical analysis and therefore critical thinking has occurred. What usually occurs is what is often referred to as a 'light bulb moment'. At this point, a student can associate and recognize the mental agility that they employ in everyday life as a transferable skill to academia. Critical analysis then becomes somewhat less of a mystery. (You will come across examples of everyday life in terms of the skills of critique and analysis later in the chapter.)

Let me give you an example that highlights the difference between the descriptive thinking and the analytical thinking that you might observe in me and my daughter. I have recently been on holiday with her to Portugal, where we spent five days experiencing Albufeira, together with my best friend and her teenage boys. We swam, we ate amazing food, we walked along beautiful beaches, we laughed, and my daughter studied for her A level mocks on her sunbed. When it comes to Instagram, I am a descriptive thinker, so I just 'dumped' most of my holiday photos on that platform with very little thought. My pictures describe my holiday. My daughter, in contrast, placed one photo of her holiday on Instagram. She applied critical thinking to this photo. She considered her audience, she considered what she wanted the photo to say, what aspect of her holiday she wanted it to represent. She questioned what it would say about her, how her friends would respond to it, even how I would respond to it. She thought about how she wanted to represent Albufeira; she wanted to encapsulate the beauty of this place in one photo. So much thinking went into that one photograph. This is critical thinking. You will do this yourself in everyday life. Critical thinking, being critically analytical, is not out of your reach.

Exercise 2.2: Critical analysis in everyday life

Think of when you have applied critical thinking or critical analysis to something in your everyday life. Jot down your thoughts. What were you curious about, what did you investigate, what questions did you ask of yourself?

This newfound understanding of critical thinking, however, is not always then transferred to reflection, whether you are reflecting for you or reflecting for your course in whatever manner you are required to reflect. When using reflective models to structure their reflections, especially in relation to reflective writing for academic assessment and presentations, some students unfortunately become *so immersed* in experience that they then provide a lengthy description of the experience they are reflecting upon, detailing how the experience made them feel. Now we know from Chapter 1 that immersion in our experience is the most important aspect of the reflective process, but to create sense-making we must push ourselves into viewing our experiences through an analytical lens. However, what often occurs when students do attempt to analyse their experience is more of an evaluation of what went well and what did not go so well, or the for-and-against of the argument.

If we take a brief look at two widely used reflective models – Gibbs' (1988) reflective cycle and Borton's (1970) framework for guiding reflective activities – we will see that both models require the person reflecting to provide a description of the event (see Figures 2.1 and 2.2).

In the case of Gibbs (1988), immersing ourselves in the experience so we can provide a description of the event and then recalling thoughts, feelings and behaviours is required. In the case of Borton (1970), the 'What?' requires us to tell the story of what happened. The problem occurs when the person reflecting isn't able to move beyond immersion in the experience and describe at length what happened – then, at length, the feelings that were experienced. A lengthy description of the experience and the feelings that arose is then presumed to be reflecting, but at this point no meaningful exploration or learning has occurred and the lengthy description of what took place keeps you in the first part of the reflective process, the story – immersion in the experience. If you refer to feedback you received on written reflective assignments, it may have been suggested that you were 'too descriptive for this level'. It is sometimes the case that our narrative is so important, and we are left to reflect on our own, that we don't know how to engage with the other aspects of the reflective process – we don't know how to move through the frameworks or models of reflection, and as a result we can use them incorrectly.

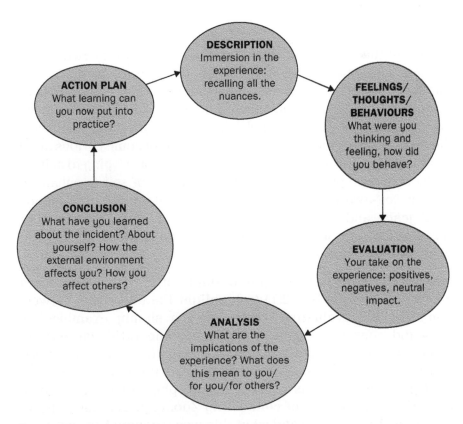

Figure 2.1 Gibbs' reflective cycle
Source: Adapted from Gibbs (1998).

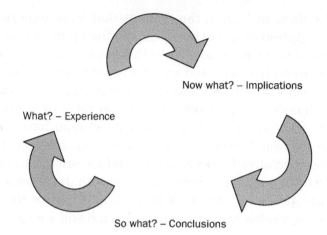

Now what? – Implications

What? – Experience

So what? – Conclusions

Figure 2.2 Borton's reflective framework
Source: Adapted from Borton (1970).

To ensure that our recollection and description of experiences can become sense-making, it is important that we apply the critical thinking that we have been discussing so far in this chapter. To learn from our story, we must understand the story and its deeper meaning. In essence, we need to apply the concept of critical analysis to the description of the experience. We need to become curious about what happened. At the end of the day, what we are trying to achieve in the reflective process is greater knowledge of self to enhance a greater self-awareness, to support the development of emotional intelligence and ultimately transformational change within ourselves and/or our practice, should change be appropriate. We want to be the *best version of ourselves*.

I would like now to show you a couple of excerpts from a student's writing (see Box 2.1) to highlight the difference between non-reflective evaluative writing, which simply examines the pros and cons in a dispassionate way, and reflective writing, where my student is really starting to apply the principles of critical thinking. You should be able to read the curiosity coming through. The student is an experienced physiotherapist bravely exploring experiences of conducting Zoom appointments during the Covid-19 pandemic and what this was teaching her about herself and her practice.

Box 2.1: Evaluative vs. reflective writing

Evaluate writing

Whilst exploring the difficulties it has forced acknowledgement that interaction with patients is poor. It has become non-responsive and almost script like. No curiosity and enthusiasm to explore the patients' needs has been demonstrated. Time constraints meant consultations occurred quickly, which was not good. There was an inability to rely on explicit and implicit non-verbal cues from the patient because of a lack of face-to-face contact and with the sudden loss of these, weaknesses in practice had been exposed. By reflecting on this, there has been recognition that active listening has not been used.

Braillon & Taiebi (2020) suggest active listening skills are easily overlooked, but they are cornerstones in communication because they foster empathy. They are simple techniques that reinforce and recognize the patient's concerns and values, creating unconditional positive regard which demonstrates concern, acceptance and understanding. Diener et al (2016) stressed active listening allows patients to express individual preferences which improves capacity for autonomous decision making. Ultimately, they influence a patient's perception of their experience and outcome of the interaction (Myers et al 2020). Further research into listening skills led to exploring empathic responding skills. Clarke (2017: 87) discusses facilitation techniques such as matching word choice and tone to the patient's emotions, reiterating, paraphrasing, and clarifying the patient's comments, whilst exploring with open questions, and offering validations and affirmations. On reflection these terms are commonly known, but not used to their full potential. These have been used inappropriately and this was affecting the way not only consultations face to face were offered but virtually during the pandemic. As a result, there is a need to review what these skills are and apply them to practice.

Reflective writing

Whilst exploring the difficulties I faced, it has forced me to acknowledge that I have become indifferent with regards interacting and communicating with patients. It has become non-responsive and almost script like. I had lost my curiosity and enthusiasm to explore the patient's needs; but why? It is easy to blame time constraints, admin, and caseload, but truthfully was it to make the consultation as quick and easy as possible? Maybe I have become complicit and presumptuous about the consultation outcome, meaning that I cut corners due to 'my experience' when ascertaining the patient's needs. Or maybe I was overly reliant on the explicit and implicit non-verbal cues from the patient and with the sudden loss of these it has exposed weaknesses in my practice. This has been difficult for me to accept about myself as a clinician. I am ashamed and upset to realize that maybe I have not been truly engaged with the patient-clinician relationship. Have I really become that apathetic and care so little? I hope not, but it suggests I have become stuck in a mindset of habitual ideologies and actions which has clouded my insight, giving me a false sense of what my 'best practice' is. By reflecting on this, I have realized the simple truth is I have not been actively listening anymore.

Are patients not fully honest with me because they do not feel heard or understood? Braillon & Taiebi (2020) suggest active listening skills are easily overlooked, but they are cornerstones in communication because they foster empathy. They are simple techniques that reinforce and recognize the patient's concerns and values, creating unconditional positive regard which demonstrates concern, acceptance and understanding. Diener et al (2016) stressed active listening allows patients to express individual preferences which improves capacity for autonomous decision making. Ultimately, they influence a patient's perception of their experience and outcome of the interaction (Myers et al 2020). Whilst researching listening skills further, I discovered empathic responding skills. Clarke (2017: 87) discusses facilitation techniques such as matching word choice and tone to the patient's emotions, reiterating, paraphrasing, and clarifying the patient's comments, whilst exploring with open questions, and offering validations and affirmations. On reflection I recognize all these terms, and they should have been embedded within my practice, but I would question how much I utilized them, either having long forgotten or ignored them. Maybe I have not embraced using them because deep down I understood I would struggle somehow. It is only after reflecting on the 'why' and identifying my communication gaps that I have moved forward.

Learning to apply these skills again has not been easy as it has necessitated a higher level of mindfulness to focus my words carefully by considering the appropriateness and outcome of my choice of words, as suggested by Bolton & Delderfield (2018). In hindsight my ambivalence to all the above has likely made my job much harder than necessary. By critically reflecting on this, I have identified that remote consultations have taught me to be more conscious about my responses rather than driven by habit. Right now, I still do not feel adept but hopefully with determination I can become an 'outstanding listener' to enable me to explore and enhance change in my patients' behaviour.

You should be able to see how the reflective writing demonstrates the student's brave curiosity and how this curiosity has pushed her into asking questions, seeking answers by examining her own behaviours and patterns, which has ultimately moved her into analytical and critical thinking. You should be able to see the connection with *self* and the difference it has made to her exploration of her experience. And you should be able to see the sense-making starting to occur so that conclusions can be drawn. Try using different coloured pens to highlight areas where you can see the curiosity, and the analysis occurring.

Now take a look at Figure 2.3, which reviews how a topic can be broken down in order to support critical analysis of that topic. The figure demonstrates how a simple topic such as a 'film review' can be broken down into its component parts (similar to mind mapping) in order to analyse the impact of the connections between the parts, and as a consequence understand how the connections impact upon the topic of a film review. All we are doing here is exploring.

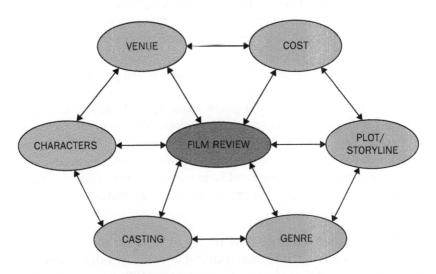

Figure 2.3 Breaking down a film review

The topic of a film review is broken down here into the parts that I might explore to help create a persuasive argument about why this is a good film. If I were to tell a friend about a film I had seen, these are the aspects I would likely discuss (not dissimilar to being a film critic). In order to now critically analyse how these parts relate to the topic, we apply intellectual curiosity to each of the parts and ask questions that help us to understand what it is about each part that helps in the process of reviewing a film. The next step is to apply intellectual curiosity to each part and question how they relate to and impact upon one another, and then question how the answers contribute to the overall impact upon the topic. If I was then *reflecting* on why this was such a good film for me, I would also explore my feelings, in combination with my thoughts: how the parts affected me, what assumptions I held about the film, how my feelings about what I had watched affected what I thought about the film and myself. I would also ask, why did I feel the way I did, how did I feel when I left the cinema, what thoughts was a I left with, where do I think these thoughts and feelings came from? What does it tell me about me? Doing this bring *us* into the critical analysis of the film review. It therefore becomes reflective.

Exercise 2.3: Film review

Imagine you are with a friend, and you are telling them about a film you have seen. Try breaking down the topic of a film review into its component parts. Ask 'what?' and 'why?' questions of each of the parts. For example, what is it about a particular part that can help you to review the film you have seen? What are the implications of that part for the topic?

Then ask yourself how all the parts relate to and impact upon one another, and how the new knowledge gained from this analysis contributes to the overall impact on your film review.

Note that the topic you choose can be anything you like: a great day out, a favourite meal, your preferred mobile phone or a favourite place. What is important at this point is the process of breaking information down.

Eventually through this process you will be able to recognize the knowledge you have, while also gaining new knowledge about yourself in relation to the topic you have chosen. What we are trying to achieve here is meaningful learning. That is, we are seeking to make sense of experiences. On making sense of what we already know (old knowledge), we gain new knowledge that can be merged with the old knowledge, which might also highlight knowledge gaps, which we can fill with research – this is often referred to as 'bridging the theory–practice gap'. This can then be used to make transformational changes to ourself and/or to our practice – that is, we become more emotionally intelligent.

Having attempted this exercise, not only should you be able to recognize which factors affect a film for you, you will also hopefully have developed a deep understanding of why certain factors are important to you and your film review. This knowledge will raise your understanding of self in relation to what films you enjoy or do not enjoy and – more importantly – why, so self-awareness is enhanced and will aid you in the future when deciding whether to view a film or not.

Having the mindset for curiosity, for interrogation, for exploration, for critical thinking is a mindset that will aid not only in reflection but in every facet of your life.

So, let's now take a look at our second essential ingredient – *knowledge*.

Knowledge

Essential ingredient #2: Knowledge

The individual, in order to analyse and reflect upon what they are experiencing in the clinical or personal setting, needs to have a level of knowledge that they can refer to and position their experience within. This knowledge enables objectivity to be brought into the subjective, filling knowledge gaps and challenging perception. If they do not have the existing knowledge, they need to know how to source the knowledge so that they may bridge that theory–practice gap and enhance their ability to understand the experience they are reflecting on.

We will now focus on what role knowledge has in supporting the reflective process and the sense-making that can occur from that critical analytical exploration of your experience.

> *'Having knowledge in all forms is amazing and powerful but*
> *having knowledge about yourself is also empowering! Having*
> *knowledge that underpins your practice in whatever guise you*
> *practise, means you can not only advocate on behalf of those*
> *you care for but on behalf of yourself!'*

When you write an academic/professional discursive essay, or are required to undertake a presentation, you will know that your arguments, statements, discussions and opinions must be created from and supported by theory and evidence in the literature, not only to lend credibility to the debate, but to demonstrate you have read deeply and widely around the subject matter, and are able to synthesize that reading into generating a discussion that helps address the topic or question at hand. You will also need to demonstrate you have engaged in meaningful research on a particular topic and that you understand what you have been reading. What is interesting is that many of my students think that the research skills they have acquired, including the ability to use the literature appropriately to create academic pieces of work, are not necessary when reflecting. As I noted previously, my students often say to me:

> *'Reflection is about me and it's personal, so why do I need to*
> *research as well?'*

In answer to this question, it is just as important to use these skills when reflecting. Evidence and literature can enhance the understanding we gain from our experiences, help determine whether our current knowledge is correct or needs to be refined, as well as help identify those gaps in our knowledge that we are not aware of. Research skills can help us determine if our tacit (assumed) knowledge is correct, current and relevant, and they can support a critique and exploration, and therefore analysis, of what we already know. The research knowledge you gain will help you raise questions about yourself, your practice and your learning. The wonderful world of literature can help bring objectivity into the subjective, challenge, confirm and add to our perceptions, help uncover unconscious bias about how we view ourselves in our experience, and enable that interrogation to take place that plays such an important role in critical thinking.

In Box 2.2 you will see how knowledge from researching and reading the literature comes into its own to help the same student we met in Box 2.1 better understand her experience through reflection. She uses some of the literature on communication and empathy to enable her to challenge her perception of self and fill those knowledge gaps about empathy which will inform her future experiences in her professional environment as a physiotherapist. The enhanced understanding obtained by applying the literature, and the increased knowledge gained when applied to her clinical practice, enables reflective practice to occur. You can see here how the knowledge gained from reading around the theme of communication and empathy has challenged the student's perception of empathy, has filled knowledge gaps and informed the practice of empathy within her future experiences with her patients.

Box 2.2: Using theory to explore and make sense of experience

With the sharp rise in social care and mental health issues experienced this year, the degree of emotional distress expressed due to isolation, lack of social support, fear, pain, and anxiety is something I have struggled with. Did I find remote consultations so difficult initially because it challenged my avoidance of the patient's emotional care needs? Maybe face-to-face I have found ways to focus elsewhere and detract or distract away from dealing with these emotional needs somehow. I recognize that I am uncomfortable having difficult conversations with patients, choosing to explore only superficial problems; but why? Honestly, selfishness plays a role, not wanting to listen, creating boundaries I do not want to cross due to fears of inadequacy about how to help. I have chosen to focus on biomedical issues and not scrutinize the psychosocial elements in depth. I always strive to show compassion to my patients, but on reflection maybe I have not always been as person-centred, authentic, or empathetic as I believed. The literature indicates empathy is important as it fosters respect, empowering the patient to exert their autonomy which deepens and nurtures the therapeutic relationship in a non-threatening and non-judgemental way (Roche & Harmon 2017). It strengthens that alliance because patients perceive they are 'being listened to' (Pinto et al 2012). Elliott et al (2011) describe empathy in clinical practice as exhibiting a compassionate attitude and willingness to sensitively understand and adopt a patient's thoughts, feelings and struggles from their point of view, and actively demonstrating that I understand their experiences. If I consider this further, Clarke (2017: 69) discusses the importance of unconditional positive regard to strengthen empathy, by suspending my own beliefs and assumptions to be able to accept the patient's values. It has saddened me to realize that maybe historically I have been judgemental and quick to dismiss these principles. I think I had forgotten the power a kind word, a listening ear or simple act of kindness can have on potentially turning a life around, and it is something that I can easily offer remotely. This insight has profoundly affected the way I now consciously choose to interact with my patients. I have learnt to embrace asking these difficult questions by putting my own fears aside, however uncomfortable it may make me feel. It is not about having an 'answer' to their problems, but about simply listening and showing understanding and acceptance of their values. I still struggle, but I hope I am now emotionally connecting more effectively to foster that mutual respect to pave the way to a stronger alliance.

Exercise 2.4: How knowledge can enhance your experience

Think of an experience you have had. Now, consider that experience and what themes might be contained within it. What theory do you think those themes are advising you to read around? What reading do you think you need to do that would help you to make greater sense of your experience.

Themes that can inform reading might be:

- Self-esteem
- Power imbalance
- Leadership
- Mentorship
- Friendship
- Family
- Growing up

Process

So how do we do this when reflecting? How are the ingredients of critical analysis and knowledge executed as part of the reflective process? Have a look at the following scenario to see these ingredients in action.

Scenario 2.1

You are a second-year student nurse/practitioner and your mentor asks you to formulate a person-centred care plan with a service user you have been spending time with during your clinical placement. Your mentor wants to assess your person-centred care planning skills.

Boxes 2.3, 2.4 and 2.5 show how old and new knowledge can be utilized during the three types of reflection – reflection pre-action, reflection-in-action, reflection-on-practice – and how critical analysis plays a role in meaningful learning.

Box 2.3: Reflection pre-action

Stage 1: Drawing on current **knowledge** of this service user, **reflect** by recalling what you think you know about them to this point. Consider both why and how you know this. Then consider your thoughts and feelings about what you know and **analyse** why you currently think and feel the way you do about this person and how you feel about undertaking the care planning session. Explore where these thoughts and feelings are emerging from and interrogate how they may affect how you behave in the care planning process. At this point, you are reflecting pre-action in a **critically analytical** manner drawing on old and current **knowledge.**

Stage 2: Consider your current **knowledge** of care planning, your current knowledge of self and of the service user.

Stage 3: Again using the skills of **critical analysis/thinking**, ask questions of your current **knowledge** in relation to what you have been asked to do, in order to understand what current **knowledge** you have and identify gaps in current **knowledge.** For example:

- Do you know what care planning is?
- Do you know how to practically undertake care planning?
- Do you know what a person-centred care plan is?
- Do you know how to be person-centred?
- Are you aware of what your current thinking and feeling are about undertaking a care plan?
- Do you have person-centred knowledge of the service user?
- Do you know what the person-centred needs of the service user are?
- Do you understand why you think and feel the way you do about this experience?
- How might you be influenced by your own culture and context, your own subjective bias, policy, procedure, status of being a student nurse – that is, being **reflexive?**

Stage 4: Gaining new **knowledge.** Take action to fill the gaps in current knowledge, e.g.

- research care planning
- speak to mentor
- observe mentor
- meet with the service user – get to know them from their own unique perspective
- research the person-centred approach
- research person-centred care planning
- practise person-centred communication skills and reflect with your mentor on your progress.

Stage 5: Acknowledge and compare new **knowledge** gained with old **knowledge.** What do you now think, and how do you now feel about being asked to undertake the care plan? Do you feel ready? You understand that the new **knowledge** either supersedes the old **knowledge** or can be assimilated and utilized harmoniously with it. At this point, a **transformational change** might take place.

Stage 6: Consider, process and **analyse** the information combined to carry out the task requested of you.

Box 2.4: Reflection-in-action

Stage 1: Begins the moment you become aware of a person-centred care plan for a service user, which might be before you meet face-to-face. You **reflect** by connecting to you and being mindful of your thoughts and feelings, and their influence on how you behave.

Stage 2: While engaging in the task requested of you, continue to **reflect** by being fully aware of your thoughts, feelings and behaviour, moment to moment, so that you can be mindful of your responses and control how they influence your responses and behaviours. Also **analyse** the way you think, feel and behave by observing the service user's responses to you and constantly checking yourself against their responses, being mindful.

Stage 3: As you **reflect**-in-action, you will realize you have some **knowledge** because you will be recalling in the moment information you need to support your engagement with the service user: you know small amounts of information about the service user, what a care plan should look like, you have likely seen a care planning session carried out by your mentor, and you know how to ask questions. You also know things about yourself.

Stage 4: It is at this point you realize you may not have the requisite **knowledge.** You may possess superficial information about the service user from a person-centred perspective. You may have very little **knowledge** about person-centred care planning and the person-centred approach. You may also perceive you do not have the knowledge to respond to the person you are caring for. You may also identify at this point why you chose not to recognize gaps in your **knowledge** prior to engaging in this experience, which you will need to explore later.

Stage 5: You could now continue formulating a potential care plan recognizing that there are fundamental gaps in your **knowledge**, knowing that the care plan process will not be proficient, but with the knowledge that your mentor/practice educator will be observing and will support you, and that the risk to self or others is minimal. Acknowledge the gaps and log these for future reference, so you can source information to fill those gaps. Acknowledge how the gaps in **knowledge** have made you feel and how this has impacted on your ability to carry out the task and as a result how it has affected your engagement with the service user. Or, you might decide to stop due to the gaps in your **knowledge**, relating this to how you feel and think and the possible effects on both you and the service user.

Stage 6: Following the experience, **reflect** and recall the gaps in your **knowledge** and take steps to fill them. Contemplate more deeply why there were gaps, why these gaps were not filled prior to the experience, and how engaging in the task with these gaps in **knowledge** felt for you. Step beyond yourself to consider how this affected the service user and how it may have felt for them – **analysis and critique.**

Stage 7: Acknowledge and compare new **knowledge** gained with old **knowledge.** You understand that the new **knowledge** either supersedes the old **knowledge** or can be assimilated and utilized harmoniously with it.

Stage 8: Reflect by considering what you have learned about yourself in this process and what this experience has taught you in relation to your personal and professional development – **analysis** and raising of self-awareness and your emotions. At this point, a **transformational change** might take place.

Box 2.5: Reflection-on-action

Stage 1: Having undertaken the person-centred care plan and having had the experience, either alone or with a friend, colleague, your mentor, personal tutor or as part of a group, **reflect** by thinking about or discussing the event in detail. This is engaging in the **reflective** process either alone or with someone else. Your **reflective** discussion will focus upon understanding your experience from your own point of view and from the point of view of the others involved. How do you think the experience went? What were your thoughts, feelings, behaviours, how do you think the service user experienced the experience? Ask 'why' and 'what' questions of what you thought/felt/behaved. Discuss or contemplate the implications of those thoughts, feelings and behaviours – **analysis**. Ask how you were influenced by your own culture and context, your own subjective bias, policy, procedure, status of being a student nurse – that is, be **reflexive**. At this point, you will have gained new **knowledge** about yourself in the context of this experience.

Stage 2: Discuss what it is you already know about person-centred care planning – **knowledge.**

Stage 3: Stages 1 and 2 will provide the framework that will support recognition that there may have been aspects of the care planning process that did not go as well as expected. Recognize that this could be because there are gaps in your current **knowledge** that hindered your ability to carry out the task in full or engendered a lack of confidence in yourself.

Stage 4: Acknowledge the gaps in your **knowledge** and take steps to fill them – **research, gain feedback**.

Stage 5: Acknowledge and compare new **knowledge** gained with old **knowledge.** You understand that the new **knowledge** either supersedes the old **knowledge** or can be assimilated and utilized harmoniously with it.

Stage 6: Reflect further by considering what you have learned about yourself in this process and what this experience has taught you in relation to your personal and professional development – **analysis.** At this point, a **transformational change** might take place.

Exercise 2.5: Now have a go!

Reflection pre-action	*Reflection-in-action*	*Reflection-on-action*
The next time you are asked to experience something that is new to you, reflect and explore the following: • What do you currently know regarding the experience you are about to have?	The next time you experience something on a placement or within the university setting (e.g. in role-play, making a cup of tea with a service user), in the moment reflect and explore:	The next time you have an experience on placement or within the university setting, reflect and explore: • What was the experience like for me? • What did I think and feel?

Reflection pre-action	*Reflection-in-action*	*Reflection-on-action*
• Do you have the full **knowledge**? • Are there gaps in your **knowledge**? • If there are gaps, fill them – **research**. • Are you confident in your ability to engage in this experience? • What are your preconceived ideas about this experience? • Will this experience tell you anything about yourself that you don't already know? • Are there things you do not know about yourself? • Where do you think these ideas and beliefs originate from and what do they mean to you? • Think about the new **knowledge** gained – can it work harmoniously with your existing **knowledge**, or does it supersede current **knowledge**? Now have the experience and think about what it might have been like had you not filled in those gaps.	• What do you already **know** about what you are currently experiencing? • What do you not **know** about what you are currently experiencing? • Is there a framework within which you could underpin the work you are doing with the individual? • Is this experience teaching you anything about yourself? • How are your thoughts, feelings and behaviours influencing you or the service user? • Has the experience highlighted any gaps in your **knowledge** that need filling? Following the experience, fill in those gaps in your knowledge and contemplate the same event had those gaps in your knowledge been filled. Would the experience have been different?	• What was the experience like for me? • What did I think and feel? • Why do I think I felt and thought in that way? • What was happening for me at the time to engender these thoughts and feelings? • How did I behave? • Why did I behave in this manner? • What impact did I have on those around me? • Has this experience highlighted any gaps in my **knowledge**? • What has this experience taught me about myself? • How do I think others experienced me and why do I think this? Now consider the gaps in your knowledge and fill them. Filling in the gaps might enable future similar events to be experienced more as you would like them to.

Now, in all three cases, ask yourself: *What do I know about myself?*

I want to share with you an example from my own experience where knowledge and sourcing information really helped me to facilitate transformational change within myself.

Many years ago, I was on the receiving end of a manager who I perceived was particularly unpleasant not just to me, but to anyone they chose to be unpleasant to. I remember having guided reflection in the form of a supervisory conversation with the wonderful mentor from when I trained as a nurse and who remained my mentor until he passed away. I remember sitting in a room crying about how awful this person was to me and how I did not know how to make it stop. I dreaded going to work. After listening to me and asking me lots of questions and acting as my sounding board, he suggested I read some literature on transactional analysis (TA). Now I am not going to go into the theoretical underpinnings of TA but suffice it to say I realized my ego state when with this person was that of a frightened child, and the individual was that of an angry adult. I read more deeply into this and using this knowledge I managed to bring some objectivity into the subjective and allow myself to explore and as a result analyse my experience differently. I amalgamated new knowledge with my current and tacit knowledge, and in the process gained greater understanding of myself. As a result, the more I read, the more I was able to explore my experiences, test out my new understanding, then explore, read more and so on and so forth. Over time, transformational change occurred within me. I grew in knowledge of myself, gained confidence, learned to behave and respond in a manner more aligned with who I actually was. I was able to finally inform my future experiences with this person to keep the interactions more productive than destructive. Remember: knowledge is powerful in a positive way.

It was the intention of this chapter to demonstrate how the two ingredients of **critical analysis** and **knowledge** play a vital role in the reflective process and your learning about you. How, by engaging in the reflective process and combining these ingredients, there is potential for you as the reflector to ultimately use the knowledge gained from reflection to generate a potential change within yourself and/or in your practice – transformational change. Let us revisit the revised extended description of reflection to see where these two ingredients are situated.

'Through a critical, analytical lens, we need to explore our experiences within the frame of how our history/background and current locus, culture and context influence who we are in our moments. Reflection requires us to open ourselves up to sourcing and learning new knowledge if the knowledge is not already known to us. And using that new knowledge gained to fill gaps in our current knowledge, challenge our preconceived notions and assumptions, and offer alternative ways of viewing experience to generate sense-making, thus creating information that can lead to personal and professional development. When we are fully open to and engaged in the process, reflection has the potential to empower us to be the best version of ourselves and inform our future experiences.'

Key points that can be taken from this chapter are:

- Critical analysis plays a key role in the reflective process.
- Critical analysis is a concept that can be applied to everyday life situations and uses skills that are transferable.
- The role of critical analysis in the reflective process is to provide a vehicle that supports exploration of an experience to empower sense-making and ensure deeper levels of learning.
- Knowledge, both old and new, plays a vital role in supporting the learning that takes place when reflecting.
- Through the reflective process we can highlight gaps in our current and tacit knowledge.
- Research plays a key part in the reflective process to support the generation of new knowledge and the learning that can occur.
- Reflection can lead to transformational change within the reflector.

CHAPTER

3

Attitudinal qualities and self-awareness

Essential ingredient #3: Attitudinal qualities

The driving force of successful engagement with the reflective process. The individual needs to be humble to the process, be open, honest and willing, having the motivation to understand and learn about themselves. The individual needs to be brave, courageous and confident in order to encourage the honesty required in the process. Offering yourself kindness, compassion and unconditional positive regard enables openness and empowers the person reflecting to connect with their authentic self.

Essential ingredient #4: Self-awareness

The individual needs to have an existing level of awareness of self, a perception of how they recognize themselves to be. It is this current knowledge of self that is the basis for exploring the self within the reflective process. Self-awareness allows the individual to be honest about how they perceive themselves to be in the experience. It is this existing knowledge of the self that is also agreed, challenged, developed and overturned in, and by, the exploration that occurs within the reflective process – leading to new knowledge of self and potential transformational change.

Learning outcomes

By the end of this chapter, you will be able to:

● Recognize the importance of the attitudinal qualities required to support being an effective reflective practitioner/person.
● Determine how you embody these qualities, recognizing those qualities you may wish to explore a deeper connection with.
● Identify how self-awareness can not only be enhanced by the reflective process but also has a vital role within the process.
● Use some of the hints and tips within this chapter to start the process of developing your own different levels of self-awareness.

Chapter 2 enabled us to explore the important roles *critical analysis* and *knowledge* play in the reflective process. I hope that you now feel comfortable with these terms and their relationship with reflection. However, as we can see from our discussion in Chapter 2 and the revised extended description of reflection given in Chapter 1, to be able to explore and challenge perception, to view our experiences through that critical analytical lens and to be open to sourcing knowledge, we require the additional ingredient that is our attitude towards ourselves and the process.

We already know reflection is about us/me/I, so to get to know us and develop differing levels of self-awareness, we need to have certain attitudinal qualities. In order to become the *best version of ourselves*, we have to commit to getting to know ourselves and then use our experiences to generate the information that will allow us to understand as much as we can about every facet of our lives. This is not, however, an easy thing to do.

The aim of this chapter, therefore, is to explore what we mean by attitudinal qualities and self-awareness, and how these are essential ingredients in helping to empower reflection. We will pay particular attention to how attitudinal qualities allow us to embrace and enhance our ability to reflect, helping us to gain levels of self-awareness that exceed what we currently have, and how having a level of self-awareness supports and enhances reflection. It is important to note that it is not the intention here to provide you with self-awareness, but to enable an understanding of why this concept is important and to provide you with hints and tips of how to start getting to know yourself.

Before we address these ingredients independently, let us briefly attempt to answer the questions in the following exercise about how our third and fourth essential ingredients – attitudinal qualities and self-awareness – intertwine. I hope that by the end of this chapter, we will have answered the questions together.

Exercise 3.1: How do the ingredients intertwine?

Read the descriptions of our third and fourth essential ingredients above. Then, jot down your answers to the following questions:

- Why do you think attitudinal qualities are important in supporting your engagement in the reflective process?
- How do you think attitudinal qualities support the gaining of self-awareness?
- Why do you think self-awareness is important in supporting your engagement in the reflective process?
- How do you think self-awareness connects and intertwines with attitudinal qualities?

Attitudinal qualities

Essential ingredient #3: Attitudinal qualities

The driving force of successful engagement with the reflective process. The individual needs to be humble to the process, be open, honest and willing, having the motivation to understand and learn about themselves. The individual needs to be brave, courageous and confident in order to encourage the honesty required in the process. Offering yourself kindness, compassion and unconditional positive regard enables openness and empowers the person reflecting to connect with their authentic self.

Before we consider the different aspects of our third essential ingredient, attitudinal qualities, let us consider what we mean by *attitude*. Early writers offered quite broad definitions of *attitude* that encompassed cognitive (thoughts), affective (emotions), motivational (enthusiasm) and behavioural (action) components. For example, Allport, a prominent writer in the field of psychology, historically defined an attitude as, 'A mental and neural state of readiness, organized through experience, exerting a directive and dynamic influence upon the individual's response to all objects and situations with which it is related' (1935: 810). Hogg and Vaughan suggested an attitude is 'a relatively enduring organization of beliefs, feelings, and behavioral tendencies towards socially significant objects, groups, events or symbols' (2005: 150). The ABC model of attitude encapsulated this quite nicely, where:

> **A** is the *affective* component, which is the emotion and feelings a person has towards something;
>
> **B** is the *behavioural* component, which is how our attitude affects how we behave towards something;
>
> **C** is the *cognitive* component, which is our beliefs, knowledge and thinking about something
>
> (Eagly and Chaiken, 1998).

Put simply, what is being suggested here is that our attitude (the way we think and feel) directs our responses (the way we behave) to the experiences that come our way.

Let us think about this in relation to the first part of the ingredient that is attitudinal qualities:

> '*The driving force of successful engagement with the reflective process. The individual needs to be humble to the process, be open, honest and willing, having the motivation to understand and learn about themselves ...*'

Here we can see that our emotions/feelings and thoughts play an important role in our wish/motivation to reflect. We can see the **A** and the **C** in play here. Connecting this first part to the reflective process, this ingredient is asking us, as the reflectors, to:

- be respectful of the process (we might just learn something!), be respectful towards ourselves when getting to know ourselves;
- recognize we could learn something (after all, do we really know everything about ourselves?);
- be enthusiastic about the potential for learning – be committed to our own development of self.

In other words, we need to *be okay with not knowing everything and be okay with getting to know ourselves in the reflective process!* If we take this on board, the **B** will enter the equation and we will then behave in a manner in the reflective process that opens the way for learning about us/me/I.

Now let us take a look at the second part of the ingredient we call attitudinal qualities:

> '*The individual needs to be brave, courageous and confident in order to encourage the honesty required in the process.*'

Ask yourself, when you started to learn about reflection, did you realize that to reflect properly you would need to be brave and honest? I can imagine your answer to be, 'no, not really!' But reflect on the following experience:

Scenario 3.1: An uncomfortable situation

You are helping your practice supervisor/practice educator to support a family whose child is in hospital. You have been left alone with the parents for a few moments while your colleague attends to another matter. The parents become upset, and you tell them everything will be okay as you perceive this to be an appropriate reassuring response. When you try to convince them that everything will all be okay, they become upset with you and raise their voices and ask you, 'how you can even know this, you don't understand how we feel'. Your practice supervisor/practice educator returns and intervenes to support the parents and the situation settles. But you internalize the parents' reaction to you and believe you have done something terribly wrong. You continue to dwell on this and worry.

The easiest option here is to ignore your feelings and thoughts and simply to continue – not to learn from the experience but to shy away from it. However, this kind of experience can remain with us.

It can inhibit our future engagement with our service users, our patients, our carers. We can become fearful of re-experiencing the situation all over again; we can become so fearful of getting it *wrong* again, we stop trying. And when a similar situation does indeed arise again, the negative feelings we experience only add to those we already had from the first situation we did not learn from. We might eventually cease to enjoy being on placement or at work, and we cease trying.

Although the above scenario might not be considered too awful or unusual an experience, if we do not process how we experienced the situation and were not to learn from it, and then experienced further uncomfortable situations that we did not reflect upon, our minor fears could develop into something more serious, something akin to the snowball effect.

So, we need to be brave. We need to have confidence in ourselves as people, and offer ourselves the kindness, compassion and care we offer to others. We need to allow ourselves to have experiences that we can learn from. We need to give ourselves permission to reflect. At this point, we need to be honest with ourselves about what we experienced, as well as honest about the feelings and thoughts we had at the time. We need to validate our narrative – that is, practise self-care (Clarke, 2022). We need to explore the experience, acknowledging what we don't know, and getting to know what we don't know so that we can fill those gaps in our knowledge. We should seek feedback from our practice supervisor or the people advising us and explore the experience with them, using their wisdom and knowledge to improve our own. We need to read the literature on communication/delivering bad news/being with people, etc. We need to be brave enough to use the feedback and literature to explore ourselves within the context of that experience so we can increase our knowledge of self, and we will learn from what occurred. By doing so, we can develop both personally and professionally. And we will grow in our confidence to reflect knowing what the process can offer us in empowering us to become the *best version of ourselves*.

Now let us take a look at the third and final part of attitudinal qualities:

> *'Offering yourself kindness, compassion and unconditional positive regard enables openness and empowers the person reflecting to connect with their authentic self.'*

The most important thing here is the reference to offering *unconditional positive regard* to ourselves. In our person-centred practice as nurses, healthcare practitioners and educators, it is expected we will be non-judgemental towards the people we care for and work with. But we don't always realize the need to apply this expectation to ourselves. So, what does this term mean? Carl Rogers, a prominent psychologist, one of the founders of humanism – a theoretical paradigm – and the founder of the person-centred approach to counselling, likened unconditional positive regard to a feeling and generation of warmth and acceptance towards, along with a prizing of, the people we care for (Rogers, 1957; Mearns and Thorne, 1988; Bozarth, 2002). We ultimately accept people for who they are, allowing them to have their own opinions, attitudes, morals and values: we do not impose ourselves upon them, but neither do we have to agree with them. We offer them kindness and compassion. But what does this mean for us?

Have you ever said to yourself, '*I must not think like that. I must not feel this way*'? What we are doing here is telling ourselves off and denying our right to think and feel a certain way for fear of being judged by others that we are different or wrong. When we do this to ourselves, we become *incongruent.* We act in a different manner to how we think and feel. We brush our thoughts and feelings to one side and try to be something we are not, without first understanding our true selves. Oh, and by the way, thoughts and feelings are like dust – if you keep sweeping dust under the carpet, it just keeps floating back out!

When we offer ourselves unconditional positive regard, we allow ourselves to accept our thoughts and feelings, we are kind to ourselves, and we don't tell ourselves off for thinking and feeling a certain way. We offer ourselves compassion through wanting to understand the nature of our thoughts and feelings. Once acceptance is allowed to occur, we can start to unpick/analyse why we think and feel the way we do. It is at this point we start to learn and gain insight into ourselves. Once understanding has occurred, we can begin to determine if change needs to take place. If we do need to change, it is on the basis of understanding and choice, not ignorance and force. This type of change is then sustainable as we have made the choice and are in control of any change that occurs.

Take a look at the following two snapshots of two different students' reflective writing. These students were writing about giving up a behaviour and exploring their experience of doing so. This was for a module I ran on substance misuse. Read the two snapshots carefully and then re-read the definition of attitudinal qualities. Then have a go at Exercise 3.2.

Scenario 3.2

A female student who gave up wearing makeup for a week felt she had failed and relapsed by wearing lip balm.

> 'The second morning and I felt dreadful; I felt physically ill. I had plans made for today and needed to go out. Normally, when I'm ill I would still put on my makeup and face the day. Not today! I did look and feel awful and had conjunctivitis. This was going to be a trying day, as I was already having negative thoughts about how people would stare at me, and I knew I was going to feel very self-conscious. I had a pub breakfast with my husband, and I was grateful not many people were in there, I didn't want people seeing me without my makeup. I chatted with the landlady but felt very conscious, particularly of my eyes. Before we set off where I would normally top up my lip-stick, I applied lip balm and a little extra moisturizer. Was I cheating? I told myself it wasn't, as my lips were dry due to my cold. On reflection I realized that this was a relapse, and I was returning to my previous behaviours. I felt really guilty. It was only my second day. How was the rest of the week going to go if I am relapsing now? However, I did acknowledge the relapse and didn't see it as a failure. But I knew I had to learn to find a way to cope with the feelings of anxiety and self-awareness about not wearing makeup by keeping calm. I carried on with my planned day feeling very conscious. I hated catching a glimpse of my reflection in the mirror because I didn't recognize myself and didn't like what I saw.'

Scenario 3.3

A male student who gave up tea and coffee for a week also felt he had failed before he had even started as he drank a cup of tea on his first day of abstaining:

'*Critical thoughts about my inability to control myself also started to arise. In turn, this generated negative emotional feelings that I would normally associate with low mood, in my body. At first, this failure seemed to me to be nothing more than a setback, a delay in my progress, a possible weakness in my character. However, when I thought about it some more, I started to think that there might be an important lesson to be learned from this initial 'failure' that might help me better understand substance misuse and abstinence. When I researched this, I found that what I had been experiencing was 'ambivalence', which, according to a school of counselling called motivational interviewing, is understood to be a central obstacle to change* [Miller and Rollnick, 2002] ...

'*I now understand this lesson in the following terms: failure to abstain should not be understood as failure, but rather as an indicator of the presence of ambivalence in the mind of the abstainer, which may be rooted in a lack of preparation at the pre-contemplation stage. Understanding my 'failure' in these terms gave me plenty to work with and allowed me to feel hopeful about future attempts. For example, on reflection it seemed clear to me that I was not fully committed to abstaining from tea or coffee and that this was due to my lack of taking the experiment seriously, and a lack of understanding and appreciation of the possibility that my tea and coffee consumption could be problematic and damaging. I clearly had some work to do in the pre-contemplation stage before I should attempt abstaining again.*'

Exercise 3.2: Who has the attitudinal qualities?

Now take a look at these two snapshots in light of the ingredient that is attitudinal qualities:

- Can you see any differences between the two?
- What are those differences?
- Who has been honest?
- Who has been brave and courageous?
- Who has really opened themselves to learning?
- Who has offered themselves unconditional positive regard?
- Who is starting to understand their thoughts and feelings?

You may see something of all these elements in both snapshots. But what you will see is that these elements are engaged with on different levels and only one of the students really tries to begin to understand their experience.

What you need to do now is to consider how the ingredient of attitudinal qualities applies to you. So, think about where you feel you are in relation to these qualities. Do you have these qualities and, if so, to what degree?

Exercise 3.3: Your current positioning in relation to the attitudinal qualities

Using the table below, jot down what you think and feel about each of the qualities. As an example, the 'open to learning' columns have been filled in for you.

- *Positioning*: Do you feel you have this quality and, if you do, to what degree?
- *Experience*: Reflect on and identity an experience you have had that would support your view. Have you had any experiences that could be used to question or disagree with your view?
- *Learning*: What do you feel you have learnt about yourself undertaking this exercise and why?
- *Development*: Have you identified areas that require developing?

Quality	Positioning	Experience	Learning	Development
Open to learning	Relatively open to learning new things. Perhaps more so in my role as student, but less so in my personal life.	I ask questions of my mentors, I spend time reading and researching topics, I get anxious on placement as I know I don't	When I am out of my comfort zone I am well aware of my lack of knowledge and this makes me want to learn.	I need to be more open to listening to and learning from others outside of being a student nurse. I need to be confident

Quality	Positioning	Experience	Learning	Development
		know an awful lot. But people who know me outside of nursing would describe me as quite opinionated.	When I think I know things, I realize that I close myself off to listening to others.	enough to recognize that I might not always be right.
Honest				
Motivated				
Brave				
Kind to myself				
Non-judgemental towards myself				

What you have done here is to reflect on your experience of where you perceive yourself to be in relation to some of the attitudinal qualities required for reflection to occur. You have considered your experiences, and to a degree you have explored yourself in relation to those experiences. As a result, some learning has occurred that you can use to inform future experiences when you need to. The result is that you are starting to become a reflective practitioner!

Self-awareness

Essential ingredient #4: Self-awareness

The individual needs to have an existing level of awareness of self, a perception of how they recognize themselves to be. It is this current knowledge of self that is the basis for exploring the self within the reflective process. Self-awareness allows the individual to be honest about how they perceive themselves to be in the experience. It is this existing knowledge of the self that is also agreed, challenged, developed and overturned in, and by, the exploration that occurs within the reflective process – leading to new knowledge of self and potential transformational change.

Have a go at the following exercise.

Exercise 3.4: Self-awareness

Write down what you think you know about yourself using the following prompts.

I would describe myself as:

Other people would describe me as:

I like:

I don't like:

I like being around people who are:

The above exercise offers a few prompts to help us to consider what we think we know about ourselves. Most of us would undertake this exercise quite simply. In general, it is not difficult to provide surface level descriptions of ourselves to another person – this is called our *self-perception* or having a basic level of self-awareness. When thinking about this in relation to reflection, it is common for students also to know exactly how they felt during a particular experience. I often hear students saying:

'I felt really anxious about ...'

'I felt really confident about ...'

In Exercise 3.4, you were asked to jot down words and statements that you perceive describe what you know about yourself – that is, *self-knowledge*. Such words and statements are a descriptive representation of what you think and feel about yourself – just like the reflective statements about feelings above. What you entered into here was an act of *describing*. This is part of the first aspect of the reflective process, of which engaging with our narrative is most important. In engaging with the first part of the reflective process, our story, our narrative, the florid description of our experience, we need to connect to who we are to be able to describe our thoughts and feelings. But what is also very important is to know *why* you described yourself the way you did in Exercise 3.4. This is a deeper level of self-awareness and a level that we must want and be open to. The attitudinal qualities of humility, honesty, openness, willingness, bravery, courage and confidence to change are key ingredients in empowering us to develop self-awareness. So, looking back at the question at the start of this chapter, we can begin to see how these two ingredients connect. These qualities are the scaffolding that supports the process of gaining a deeper understanding of what lies behind your self-perception descriptors, and which will ultimately enhance your self-awareness.

Let us now make sure we understand what the term 'self-awareness' means. Eckroth-Bucher defined self-awareness as 'the cerebral exercise of introspection. This attribute reflects the cognitive exploration of own thoughts, feelings, beliefs, values, behaviours, and the feedback from others' (2010: 297). In other words, self-awareness is the thoughtful consideration of oneself. Not just self-indulgently thinking of oneself, but making a conscious effort to understand and know your own identity, beliefs, thoughts, traits, motivations, feelings and behaviours, and to recognize how these can impact on you and on those around you. Hofstadter (2007) associated self-awareness with consciousness. In developing this notion, we can say self-awareness is about recognizing we are conscious, we exist, and in that recognition we know we can think about our thoughts and actions and how we affect and influence others. Luft and Ingham (1955), two prominent psychologists, devised the Johari Window (see Figure 3.1) as a way of illustrating the concept of self-awareness.

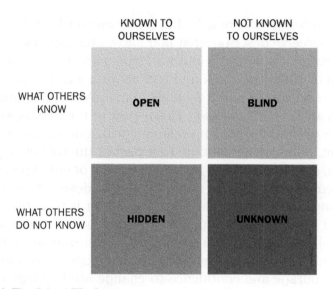

Figure 3.1 The Johari Window
Source: Adapted from Luft and Ingham (1955).

The Johari Window comprises four quadrants:

1   The *Open* quadrant signifies what you know about yourself and is also known to those around you.
2   The *Blind* quadrant represents those things other people feel they know about you, which perhaps you do not know about yourself.
3   The *Hidden* quadrant recognizes there are things you know about yourself that others do not.
4   The final quadrant is classed as *Unknown*, things that neither yourself nor other people know about you.

Our aim in the reflective process is to make the *Open* quadrant the largest quadrant. The larger it is, the more knowledge of self we have, which enables us to enhance our self-awareness further. That is not to say that you can't keep some things to yourself (*Hidden*); there may be some things about yourself that you may consciously choose not to tell others – this is okay. It is also important to note that the *Unknown* doesn't always have to remain unknown. You may have had an experience that tells you something quite surprising about yourself that neither you nor others were aware of. What is most important here is opening yourself up to getting to know your *Unknown* areas.

You also need to understand that our *Blind* area can diminish through the reflective process by encouraging feedback from others to support the expansion of our *Open* quadrant. Remember, when trying to enhance self-awareness we are trying to gain more knowledge of what constitutes *I*, as it is this knowledge of self that allows us to then explore ourselves in the context of use.

If you consider Exercise 3.4 in relation to the Johari Window, what you did was to reveal your *Open* and maybe also aspects of your *Hidden* quadrant. So let's now see how much you understand these factors about yourself. Have a go at completing Exercise 3.5.

Exercise 3.5: What is your level of self-awareness? Let's reflect on the experience of describing *I*!

Take another look at Exercise 3.4 and ask yourself questions about each of the things you described.

● Why would you describe this aspect as being part of who you are?
● What evidence do you have?
● What impact does this aspect have on you?
● What impact does this aspect have on those around you? What feedback have you received?
● How functional is this aspect of you? How well do you utilize this aspect of you? Does it work for you?
● What evidence do you have to support the functionality or non-functionality of this aspect?
● Do you need to modify this aspect?
● Is this how you want to describe yourself or be known as?

To answer these questions to the best of your ability, you need to connect with the 'attitudinal qualities' ingredient. So, to answer these questions to heighten your self-awareness, you need to be open, honest, brave and non-judgemental about yourself. It is very hard to be honest with ourselves when we judge ourselves for who we are. What you are doing here is connecting the ingredient of attitudinal qualities with the ingredient of self-awareness.

By looking at our fourth essential ingredient, self-awareness, we will see that we need a certain level of self-awareness to be able to reflect.

> *'The individual needs to have an existing level of awareness of self, a perception of how they recognize themselves to be. It is this current knowledge of self that is the basis for exploring the self within the reflective process. Self-awareness allows the individual to be honest about how they perceive themselves to be in the experience. It is this existing knowledge of the self that is also agreed, challenged, developed and overturned in, and by, the exploration that occurs within the reflective process – leading to new knowledge of self and potential transformational change.'*

Atkins and Murphy (1993) believed that self-awareness is the foundation skill upon which reflection and reflective practice are built. In essence, to be able to reflect, *you need to know yourself* to some degree. It enables you to see yourself in a particular situation and honestly observe how you have affected that situation and how the situation has affected you. It further allows you to analyse your feelings regarding that particular experience, as the self-awareness you currently have ensures you already know what your thoughts and feelings are. Self-awareness is central to the ability to be self-critical, self-directing and self-motivated (Smith, 2011). If we look at this in relation to being a nursing student/healthcare practitioner/educator, having a level of self-awareness when caring for or looking after more vulnerable people allows you to recognize what your own value systems are and know that they may be different to the person you are caring for or supporting. It allows you to put these value systems to one side in order to understand the value systems of the person you are looking after.

To be able to learn from the reflective process, therefore, you need to be able to get to know yourself at a deeper level. However, developing this deeper level of honest self-awareness is not easy. Our current level of self-awareness may not be altogether fully unbiased. Atkins (2004) recognized that individuals have a tendency to want to portray themselves in a favourable light or in a positive frame – at the end of the day, who doesn't want people to see them as inherently good? However, it is this natural human tendency that can interfere with our ability to reflect objectively and ultimately gain that deeper understanding. In light of this, you will now see why the ingredient of attitudinal qualities –honesty, bravery, and so on – plays such a vital role not only in reflection and reflective practice, but in gaining the deeper levels of self-awareness that we need to be able to learn about ourselves and develop as practitioners and as people. It is having the attitudinal qualities required for the reflective process that helps remove our biased view of ourselves and opens us up to learning: 'It takes considerable time, effort, determination, courage and humour to initiate and maintain effective reflection' (Taylor, 2006: 48).

Let us consider what we have learnt so far. We know that our attitude plays a vital role in being able to reflect effectively and to take on board the learning that can occur from successful reflection. Some of the exercises in this chapter have been designed to enable you to begin to understand your own attitudinal qualities and highlight areas for your attitudinal development. We have seen that reflection generates self-awareness, but ironically, we do need a level of self-awareness in order to reflect successfully in the first place! All of the exercises in this chapter will support you in generating greater levels of self-awareness.

Now let's review what these exercises are asking us to do when getting to know ourselves. Have a go at completing Exercise 3.6.

Exercise 3.6: Generating self-awareness. Let us reflect on experience!

The nature of the experience	Thoughts	Ask yourself
What happened? What were you involved in? Who was with you at the time?	Identify one thought you had that stands out for you as important.	• Why have I chosen this thought to reflect on? • What happened at the time to make me think this? • Why did I think this? • Did what happen justify my thought?

The nature of the experience	Thoughts	Ask yourself
		• What values of mine do I believe made me think this way? • Was my thought influenced by anything else at the time – things, people? • What was the impact of that thought on my behaviour? • How did that thought make me feel at the time? • What impact did how I felt have on me at the time? • How did this affect me following the experience? • What do I feel I have learned about myself? • How was this thought influenced by others? • How did this thought influence any other person in my experience?

We can determine from this exercise that all we are doing is asking lots of questions about the nature of our experiences and then trying to answer them. The questions posed in this exercise are designed to probe quite deeply into our thoughts, but we can use the same or similar questions to probe deeply into our feelings and behaviours in the hope that the answers we give to ourselves will generate some knowledge of self that we can assimilate and use in the future. We are simply trying to get to know ourselves.

We can also undertake the same exercise in relation to the *Blind* quadrant of the Johari Window. Remember that the *Blind* quadrant is where others may know something about us that we do not. However, what others know can become known to us if we are open to learning – these aspects do not need to stay blind forever. A person we have come into contact with – a family member, mentor, friend, partner, boss – may choose to tell us something about ourselves we were unaware of. It could be how we come across to people in certain situations, how we make someone feel without realizing it, or it may be how we have responded to a person in our care. This does not always need to be a negative observation.

So now have a go at completing Exercise 3.7 and see if you can make something that sat in the *Blind* quadrant part of the *Open* quadrant.

Exercise 3.7: Generating self-awareness. Let us explore the *Blind* quadrant!

The nature of the experience	Thoughts	Ask yourself
Recall an experience when someone told you something about you that you were unaware of. What happened? Who told you? What were you involved in? Who was with you at the time?	What was the person's observation, thought, feeling about you? What did they tell you about yourself you did not know already?	• Why have I chosen this to reflect on, and what is the significance of this? • What happened at the time to make them highlight this to me? • What was my reaction to them on telling me? • What was I doing in order to make them see me in this light? • What values of mine do I believe made me behave this way? • Was my behaviour influenced by anything else at the time – things, people? • How do I feel about what they told me? • What do I think about what they have told me? • What was the impact of what they told me on my future behaviour, thoughts, feelings? • Do I agree with their observations about me? • What do I feel I have learned about myself?

To recap, all we have been doing in the exercises in this chapter is to reflect on experiences. We have diligently considered our experiences, asked lots of questions and answered them.

It was the intention of this chapter to demonstrate how the two ingredients of attitudinal qualities and self-awareness play a vital role in the reflective process. We have seen how they support each other and, if combined effectively, allow us to gain deeper levels of understanding about the person we are and thus raise our levels of emotional intelligence. We can see how by engaging in the reflective process and combining these ingredients, we can develop as unique individuals with higher levels of self-awareness that will help to support and enhance our clinical and professional practice.

If we revisit the extended description of reflection, we can see where these two ingredients are situated:

> *'Then stepping beyond the self and using this knowledge gained to understand how we may then have influenced those around us. To be fully immersed in this process, we must be open to learning about what constitutes 'I', leaving arrogance and complacency at the door, be kind and compassionate enough to offer ourselves unconditional positive regard, be actively engaged in mindfulness, and consciously aware of the self in our moments.'*

Key points that can be taken from this chapter are:

- Attitudinal qualities play a vital role in ensuring effective, successful reflection occurs.
- Attitudinal qualities support our ability to become self-aware.
- A level of self-awareness is required to reflect.
- Reflection can generate much deeper levels of self-knowledge that can then be used to enhance self-awareness.
- We need to be open to understanding ourselves.
- High self-awareness and the right attitude can engender good clinical and professional practice, as we understand ourselves in the context of others.

Being person-centred and being empathic

Essential ingredient #5: Being person-centred

The person reflecting has vast resources for self-understanding. These resources for self-understanding can be accessed if we are person-centred with ourselves. Recognizing we have our own unique subjective view of the world (our individual phenomenology) allows us to create a climate whereby we can get to know ourselves and gain a deeper understanding of ourselves in relation to our experiences. With understanding, a heightened level of self-awareness grows. We are able to develop both personally and professionally.

Essential ingredient #6: Being empathic

The person reflecting needs to want to understand themselves in relation to their experiences accurately. They need to use the skills of empathic questioning and responding to allow for deeper analysis and as a result understanding and sense-making of their thoughts, feelings and behaviour in relation to the experience they are reflecting on. Not only this, they need also to be able to use their empathy to understand how others perceive them and the experience they have been part of.

Learning outcomes

By the end of this chapter, you will be able to:

● Appreciate the importance of being person-centred and how it supports successful reflection.
● Explore how person-centred you are with yourself and be able to recognize areas where you need to be more person-centred.
● Utilize the concept of empathy when moving through the reflective process.
● Use the knowledge gained to be person-centred and empathic with yourself in the reflective process.

In Chapter 3, we discussed the vital role that *attitudinal qualities* and *self-awareness* play in the reflective process. We acknowledged that in order to get to know ourselves at a deeper level in the process, we need to have the attitudinal qualities (such as courage, bravery and openness) required for the learning about ourselves to take place, and so gain that greater level of self-understanding. The revised extended description of reflection discussed in Chapter 1 also asks us to become our own person-centred enquirer, recognizing the need for us to understand ourselves empathically and accurately. Being our own person-centred enquirer, using empathy to support understanding of self, is not possible without applying everything we discussed in Chapter 3 regarding our attitude towards ourselves and the reflective process.

> Registered nurses act in the best interests of people, putting them first and providing nursing care that is person-centred, safe and compassionate.
>
> (NMC, 2018a: 7)

The Nursing and Midwifery Council (NMC) has recognized the importance of being person-centred by embedding the notion into their updated Code of Conduct (NMC, 2018b) for nurses and midwives and their Standards of Proficiency for Registered Nurses (2018a). The Health & Care Professions Council have also embedded person-centred care into their Standards for Proficiency (HCPC, 2023). So, we know it is important to embody and apply being person-centred within our practice, but I imagine this is not a notion you might naturally apply to yourself.

In this chapter, we are going to take a more in-depth look at the notion of being person-centred. We will not look in detail at how it relates to care, as this you will learn in your training; instead, we will look at how it supports you in getting to know yourself and as a result enables and supports the reflective process. By really trying to understand what the notion of being person-centred means in relation to reflection, you will, as a result, develop a better idea of what it means for care and clinical practice. We will also take a close look at empathy. Empathy is a fundamental part of being person-centred, as we shall see in this chapter, and is a term that even seasoned practitioners sometimes misunderstand. Empathy is also in my opinion one of the most important concepts for us as practitioners to understand. It underpins all types of therapeutic communication and ensures we understand our patients and the people we support from their own unique perspective and to a degree that supports person-centred practice.

I hope, therefore, having completed this chapter, you will be able to identify how all the knowledge we gained from Chapter 3 applies here and how the notions of person-centredness and empathy are inextricably intertwined.

So, let us now take a look at our fifth essential ingredient – *being person-centred*.

Being person-centred

Essential ingredient #5: Being person-centred

The person reflecting has vast resources for self-understanding. These resources for self- understanding can be accessed if we are person-centred with ourselves. Recognizing we have our own unique subjective view of the world (our individual phenomenology) allows us to create a climate whereby we can get to know ourselves and gain a deeper understanding of ourselves in relation to our experiences. With understanding, a heightened level of self-awareness grows. We are able to develop both personally and professionally.

Although I have advised we will not be looking in detail at person-centred care, I do want to touch upon something we discussed in the first edition of this book to re-highlight how person-centred care is linked with reflection and the need for us to be person-centred within the reflective process. The person-centred nursing framework developed by McCormack and McCance (2006, 2010) and further discussed by Dewing et al. (2021) comprises four domains:

- the attributes of the nurse – *prerequisites*;
- the environmental context – *the care environment*;
- the processes that support being person-centred in care – *care processes*; and
- patient outcomes – *person-centred outcomes*.

What I wish to focus on is the first domain, the *prerequisites* of the nurse. To be able to provide effective person-centred care, Dewing et al. go beyond the nurse requiring knowledge and skill to be competent and focus on the *knowing of self* and *clarity of beliefs and values*:

> Knowing self:
> The way a nurse makes sense of his/her knowing, being and becoming a person-centred practitioner through reflection, self-awareness, and engagement with others.
>
> Clarity of beliefs and values:
> The awareness of the impact of nurses' beliefs and values on the care experience provided by nurses and the commitment to reconcile beliefs and values in ways that facilitate person-centredness.
>
> (2021: 17)

Here we can clearly see the authors wishing to make the connection with how self-awareness, knowing who we are in the context of others, enables effective person-centred care. In order to truly understand another from their own unique perspective, we have to know who *we* are, so we do not transpose our own vision for what we want onto those we care for.

Have a go at the following exercise.

Exercise 4.1: Being person-centred

Consider your own understanding of the term 'being person-centred'. Write down what this term means to you, in relation to your practice and what you think it means in the reflective process. We will come back to this at the end of the chapter to see if you come to view the notion differently once you have worked through the chapter.

- I understand 'being person-centred' in relation to my practice to mean ...
- I understand 'being person-centred' in relation to when I reflect to mean ...

The way in which I want you to understand the notion of being person-centred for the purposes of reflection requires me to introduce one of the most influential psychologists of all time, Carl Rogers (Kirschenbaum and Henderson, 1989: xiii). Rogers, one of the founders of humanistic psychology and the founder of the person-centred approach to counselling, developed his own theory of personality and counselling. Unlike some counselling schools of thought, he believed that the counsellor should not simply adopt a set of tools and techniques for helping someone but adopt instead a *way of thinking and behaving* towards the individual requiring help.

Rogers believed that the helper has an attitude that consumes and, in simple terms, embodies the way they think, feel and act towards another individual. It is these attitudinal qualities that provide the orientating framework within which the counsellor, helper or nurse views the world. Rogers referred to this attitude as a way of 'being' and was clear that the person-centred therapist, nurse or helper could be an imperfect person-centred practitioner as long as they did not perceive the approach as solely a set of techniques (Rogers, 1951). Rogers was clear that in order to help another individual, one cannot make assumptions about what they are experiencing, thinking and feeling; as a helper, we need to accurately understand the person we are helping and, in accurately understanding them, we can help them to understand themselves. The approach takes a non-directive stance, it doesn't look to solve people's problems for them, and it recognizes people as their own experts (Rogers, 1951). Rogers believed that by embracing the person-centred approach, the practitioner would allow their personality to shine through – that is, be transparent and congruent. Take another look at what you wrote down for Exercise 4.1. Does anything mentioned here align with what you wrote about what you understand being person-centred to mean in your practice? If it doesn't, try to determine why and what gaps in your knowledge you need to fill through further reading.

Now, what does this mean in relation to reflection and what does being person-centred mean when we apply it to ourselves in the reflective process? Being person-centred with ourselves in the reflective process means that we wish to understand accurately how we think and feel about our own experiences. My own understanding of reality comes from understanding my subjective interpretation of the things I experience. Understanding the world and understanding me is about understanding what 'I' believe exists. We will not assume to know what we think and feel, or try and interpret why we think, feel and behave the way we do. We are not going to tell ourselves how we should think and feel either. We just want to understand ourselves accurately. As a result, we shall get to know ourselves.

It is not my intention here to provide you with a theoretical lecture on Rogers' philosophy of therapy. Rather, it is to understand the central assumption of Rogers' person-centred approach as it relates to reflection, which can be briefly stated as follows:

> It is that the individual has within himself or herself vast resources for self-understanding, for altering his or her self-concept, attitudes and self-directed behaviour – and that these resources can be tapped if only a *definable climate of facilitative psychological attitudes can be provided.*
>
> (Rogers, 1980: 115–16, original emphasis)

Applying this statement from Rogers to the reflective process, what we are interested in is the part that is not in italics. In embodying what it is to be person-centred, we know that we have the ability to understand ourselves and from learning about ourselves we can fundamentally alter the way we then act in the world, although Rogers talks about this only happening if we provide the right climate for ourselves to grow and develop. It is this *climate* underpinning being person-centred, providing the framework for the reflective process, that we will look at closely in this chapter.

Consider this idea of providing a *climate*.

Exercise 4.2: The climate for change

Jot down what aspects/factors would need to be present when talking to another person in order for you to be open and honest about how you feel and think.

Rogers (1957) originally proposed that six conditions need to exist for change to occur within a person. It is these six conditions that he suggested provide the climate for change. In the reflective process, for you to get to know yourself and allow change for the better to occur, you need to embody the six conditions shown in Box 4.1 and apply them.

Box 4.1: The six necessary and sufficient conditions for therapeutic change

1   A client and a helper are in psychological contact.
2   The client sees him or herself in need of help.
3   The helper is congruent and genuine.
4   The helper experiences unconditional positive regard towards the client in need of help.
5   The therapist experiences an empathic understanding of the client's internal frame of reference and endeavours to communicate this experience to the client.
6   The communication to the client of the therapist's empathic understanding and unconditional positive regard is to a minimal degree achieved.

Source: Adapted from Rogers (1957).

Have a look at the conditions in Box 4.1. How does what you jotted down compare with the conditions in the box?

If you are at all familiar with Rogers' work, you may have come across the notion of the *three core conditions* (Figure 4.1). Over time, the six conditions for therapeutic change were simplified and combined – to become the three core conditions – by supporters of the person-centred philosophy. There are some who would criticize this simplification and suggest that this reduction has resulted in the misunderstanding that the therapeutic relationship within the person-centred framework is about 'doing to' rather than 'being with' the patient (Sanders, 2006). But for our purposes of using this approach within the reflective process, the three core conditions provide a very useful climate within which we can safely get to know ourselves. So, let's take a closer look at the three core conditions and see how they enable us to be person-centred with ourselves, creating the climate within which to reflect openly and honestly.

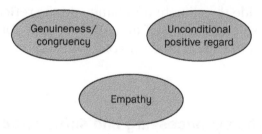

Figure 4.1 The three core conditions

Since I view empathy as such an important condition, it is treated here as one of the ten essential ingredients for successful reflection, and as a result I will address empathy in the second part of this chapter. But let us first look at the other two core conditions in this model, the concepts of (1) genuineness/congruency and (2) unconditional positive regard.

Genuineness and congruency

Exercise 4.3: Exploring genuineness and congruency

Jot down what you think 'being genuine and congruent' means. First, consider the general meaning of being genuine and congruent. Then, consider what it would mean in relation to you when reflecting. Finally, consider what it would mean when applied in the helping relationship with another person.

Let us consider this core condition in a little more detail before we review your own understanding in light of the new information.

Rogers proposed two meanings for this notion of being genuine and congruent. The first meaning relates to his patients coming to him for help in the counselling relationship. In this instance, being congruent means that our non-verbal and verbal behaviours towards another align with our genuine thoughts and feelings. So, for example, if you don't understand what the person you are caring for is trying to say, you shouldn't tell them that you do. Instead, you should verbalize that you are not clear as to what they mean and help them to explain in greater depth so you do eventually understand. The second relates to the person helping and their state of mind. We are also interested in this second meaning, since it relates to us in the helping relationship we have with ourselves when reflecting:

> The therapist should be, within the confines of this relationship, a congruent, genuine integrated person. It means that within the relationship the person is freely and deeply himself, with his actual experience accurately represented by his awareness of himself.
>
> (Rogers, 1957: 97)

Let's simplify this. What this means for us in the relationship we have with ourselves in the reflective process is that we are open to ourselves. We are honest with ourselves about what we have experienced. We allow ourselves to be honest about how we think and feel about what we are experiencing, and we don't try to be something we are not. We are real and authentic.

How many times have you said to yourself?

'I can't think like that. I mustn't feel this way.'

How helpful are we being to ourselves if we are not genuine and real about what we think and feel? The only way to understand ourselves is to be ourselves in the reflective process, not what we think others or society expects us to be. To understand this more clearly, let us briefly consider what this means in the helping relationship towards another person.

Take a look at Figure 4.2. When you *act* the role of the nurse, when you put up a professional façade, the person you are helping will try and connect with you but won't be able to because the acting role will stop them from accessing you as a person. The rectangle in the figure represents the barrier that is created when you act the part, rather than allow your own personality to come through. As a helper, you should be confident enough in yourself that you allow yourself to be a real, authentic person with the individuals you are trying to help.

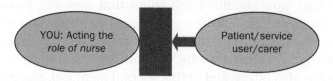

Figure 4.2 Acting the role of nurse – lacking genuineness and congruency

Let us now consider this in relation to a person who is about to have an operation on their knee to repair a torn anterior cruciate ligament (ACL) and who is being care for by an operating department practitioner (ODP) in the pre-operative phase prior to anaesthesia.

Patient: '*I am terrified, I hate hospitals, don't they scare you?*'

The ODP who is confident enough in him or herself to be authentic and transparent might respond in the following way:

ODP: '*Honestly, no I do not get scared now as I am a very used to operating theatres, so I don't fully understand your fear as I am comfortable here, but I am aware you are scared right now. Is there anything I can do to help ease some of your fear?*'

Here the ODP has been congruent. They have been respectfully honest with the patient; they have been real and authentic with compassion and kindness. The patient can connect with this ODP.

As you can see from Figure 4.3, when the nurse embodies the notion of genuineness and congruency no barriers are present, the service user can connect and the therapeutic relationship can now develop. The service user doesn't access the whole of the nurse, but the nurse's transparency allows the service user to view the nurse as a real person with thoughts and feelings of their own, not a cardboard cut-out of what they think a nurse should be.

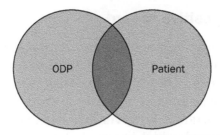

Figure 4.3 When genuineness and congruency are present

So, let's relate this to the reflective process. If when you are reflecting you are honest with yourself, congruent and real about what you are or have thought and felt, you can access yourself and therefore gain a greater understanding of yourself.

Now take a look at Figure 4.4. Here, the two interconnecting circles represent the reflective process. The circles demonstrate how, by embodying the core condition of genuineness and congruency, you are able to access and get to know yourself to the extent represented by the overlap of the circles.

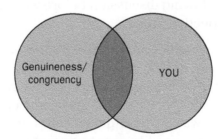

Figure 4.4 Accessing yourself in the reflective process

Eventually, as you become more confident in being really honest with yourself, allowing yourself to be fully you when reflecting, there will only be a single circle, as you will be fully accessible to yourself. You can perhaps start to see now why what we discussed in Chapter 3 in relation to those attitudinal qualities is so important for this ingredient.

Now that we understand the core condition of *genuineness*, let's take a look at the core condition of *unconditional positive regard*.

Unconditional positive regard

Unconditional positive regard has been a source of contention within the literature for several years – possibly prior to and certainly since Rogers in both his key papers stated: 'That the therapist is experiencing unconditional positive regards toward the client' (Rogers, 1959: 213). Its importance, however, has been noted by the Nursing and Midwifery Council, which states that as nurses, 'You make sure that those receiving care are treated with respect, that their rights are upheld and that any discriminatory attitudes and behaviours towards those receiving care are challenged' (NMC, 2018b: 6).

Have a go now at the following exercise.

Exercise 4.4: Defining unconditional positive regard

Using your knowledge to date, jot down your understanding of unconditional positive regard.

Now consider your understanding of unconditional positive regard in relation to the following discussion before we contemplate how it is helpful in the reflective process.

Rogers perceived unconditional positive regard to be a warm acceptance of each aspect of the client's experience. Taking this into account, in order to offer unconditional positive regard, we need to recognize and accept every aspect of the person coming for help for who they are, with warmth and genuineness and without judging them. Furthermore, we need to recognize that they will need, eventually, to be able to understand themselves clearly, but before this can happen they need to accept themselves holistically. It is thought that offering unconditional positive regard supports acceptance on behalf of the person coming for help so that they can gain greater self-awareness (Dexter and Wash, 2001).

It is the suspension of our own beliefs, ideas and assumptions that underpins our ability to offer unconditional positive regard and, as a result, accept the person in need of help for who they are. In accepting the person in need of help for who they are, they will be able to begin to accept themselves.

However, it is important to note here that accepting the client for who they are and not judging them or offering an opinion does not mean that you agree with that person's beliefs, values or behaviour. When I discuss this notion of unconditional positive regard with my nursing students, the thought of acceptance and suspending one's personal judgements tends to create uncertainty and the impression that it also means agreeing with or condoning behaviour. However, this is not the case and, as already stated, *acceptance and being non-judgemental does not mean you are in agreement.* Is this what you first considered unconditional positive regard to be? How does this compare with what you jotted down when completing Exercise 4.4?

Our next question is how does unconditional positive regard relate to the reflective process? As you will be aware from the previous chapters, reflection is about gaining greater self-awareness by getting to know ourselves in the reflective process. The offering of unconditional positive regard towards ourselves when we reflect, accepting ourselves for who we are, and not judging ourselves in relation to our thoughts and feelings, allows us to feel accepted without being judged by the person most important to us – ourselves. As a result, we may feel free to be truly honest about our own thoughts and beliefs without fear of condemnation in the reflective process. By not judging ourselves, we can be truly honest and as a result get to know and understand ourselves at a deeper level.

Let's take another look at the aspects of the ingredient that is being person-centred. Can you see how unconditional positive regard connects to this ingredient?

> '*These resources for self-understanding can be accessed if we are person-centred with ourselves. Recognizing we have our own unique subjective view of the world (our individual phenomenology) allows us to create a climate whereby we can get to know ourselves and gain a deeper understanding of ourselves in relation to our experiences. With understanding, a heightened level of self-awareness grows. We are able to develop both personally and professionally.*'

And if we take another look at one aspect of the ingredient of attitudinal qualities from Chapter 3, we can see its relevance here too:

> *'Offering yourself kindness, compassion and unconditional positive regard enables openness and empowers the person reflecting to connect with their authentic self.'*

Take a look now at Scenario 4.1 and see unconditional positive regard in action.

Scenario 4.1

This female student is reflecting on her experiences of the caring process as a mental health nurse, looking after a pregnant drug user. She has allowed herself to be truly honest about what she thinks and how she feels. Ultimately, this will allow her to understand and accept herself, giving meaning to the learning taking place.

> *'My interactions also showed an element of co-dependency, I felt that if I was good enough, I could change her behaviour, not acknowledging that change has to come from within. I made decisions based upon what I thought Mary wanted me to do. I had created a dependent relationship, subconsciously perhaps to replace the dependency I had lost from my own daughter, and the dilemma now was if I discouraged this dependency would I be viewed as a loved mother, disapproving but now rejecting mother, perpetuating her lifelong cycle of rejection and hopelessness.*
>
> *'I found my feelings regarding this transference and counter-transference to be very intense, agreeing with Ryum et al. (2010), who suggest that such reactions can provoke greater anxiety for both the client and professional, that transference and counter-transference can either impede the therapeutic relationship or provide an increased level of empathy.'*

Let's now take a look at the sixth essential ingredient – *being empathic.*

Being empathic

Essential ingredient #6: Being empathic

The person reflecting needs to want to understand themselves in rela-
tion to their experiences accurately. They need to use the skills of
empathic questioning and responding to allow for deeper analysis and
as a result understanding and sense-making of their thoughts, feelings
and behaviour in relation to the experience they are reflecting on. Not
only this, they need also to be able to use their empathy to understand
how others perceive them and the experience they have been part of.

An integral part of being person-centred is the notion of empathy –
embodying what it means to be empathic will support our endeavour to
accurately understand ourselves within a person-centred framework.
Empathy is one of the most important ingredients to support understanding not only of yourself in the reflective process, but also
understanding your service users in the person-centred caring process. The good news here is that empathy is strengthened by the first
two core conditions of genuineness and unconditional positive regard
that we have already discussed in relation to the fifth essential ingredient – that of being person-centred. Without these two conditions
being in place, we cannot truly be empathic. As such, the first thing
we need to acknowledge is that in being empathic we combine and
embody two components of attitude and skill. It is my belief that in
being truly empathic, we cannot have one without the other.

To be truly empathic, we need to embody the attitude of empathy,
which is 'I am a transparent, accessible person with a genuine interest in the person I am caring for or supporting', or as in the case of
reflection, a genuine interest in wanting to really get to know you. In
other words, this attitude is an amalgamation of the first two core
conditions in the person-centred framework. The second thing to
consider is that empathy is also a skill set. The skills of empathic
responding, which will be addressed in full in Chapter 5, combined
with the right attitude, will enable the empathic process to be useful
and to be experienced positively by the person you are caring for or
by yourself when reflecting.

So, before we go any further and acknowledge some of the skills of empathic responding, we need to consider carefully what we mean by being empathic. Have a go at the following exercise.

Exercise 4.5: Defining empathy

Again using the knowledge that you have, how would you define empathy?

When I ask my students what they think empathy is, they often respond as follows:

> '*Trying to view and see the world through someone else's eyes, then imagining what it would be like if it was me.*'

> '*Trying to imagine what someone is going through.*'

Now keep these quotes in mind as we learn a little bit more about empathy and whether my students had an accurate understanding of this concept.

Empathy has been widely discussed in the literature and several authors would acknowledge empathy has having three levels. The first level is often classed as *affective empathy* or *emotional contagion*. This is where, for instance, you are in a room full of students who are laughing and you can't help but laugh along with them. This level of empathy is the most basic and requires no understanding on your behalf as to why the group are laughing.

The next level of empathy has become a concept all on its own. This second level is when we experience concern, sorrow or sadness for another person (Wispé, 1986); we don't understand their feelings and thoughts, yet we assume to know how the person is experiencing their reality. As a result, this has been termed *sympathy* and is considered a separate entity to that of empathy, and so needs to be understood differently.

The final and most complex level of empathy is that with which we are most interested – that level of empathy when cognition (thinking) comes into play. Here, there is an appreciation of the feelings experienced by another, and an understanding of the other's internal world. This understanding is then communicated back to the other person (Rogers, 1967), who perceives this empathy and uses it as a way of gaining greater self-understanding (Nelson-Jones, 2006). Rogers suggested that in being empathic, you experience these feelings as if they are your own. But you never lose the 'as if' quality and never lose a sense of self. Empathy is a dynamic affective (emotional) and cognitive (thoughtful) complex process. Our aim as nurses and helpers when being empathic is to accurately understand how another person is experiencing their world without making assumptions. Being self-aware as we have previously discussed assists us in suspending our own assumptions and judgements so that we can really try to understand another from their own internal frame of reference (Rogers, 1967; Brammer and MacDonald, 1996). The communication skills discussed in the next chapter will support and enable you to be empathic.

Now take a look at Exercise 4.6.

Exercise 4.6: Empathy vs. sympathy

A friend of yours is telling you how she feels about separating from her partner. She has concerns about being isolated – she is now a single parent and feels a sense of loss of role as she is no longer 'the other half'. She is excited about what the future might hold for her because she perceived having been controlled by the other person in the relationship. She also feels ashamed as this is not what she had expected for her family; she feels broken.

Take a look at this first possible interaction between you and your friend:

> Friend: *'I feel awful since they walked away, I feel so sad and empty. I am really worried.'*

> You: *'Oh I am so sorry to hear they left, I know how you feel, and I felt exactly the same when I split up with my other half last year. I was really worried I would be on my own forever.'*

Now have a go at answering the following questions in relation to the response:

- What do you think you may have been feeling towards your friend?
- Why do you think you responded in this manner? Which of the six necessary and sufficient conditions for therapeutic change do you think you are demonstrating here? (see Box 4.1)
- What type of a response is this – empathic or sympathetic?
- How do you imagine your friend is likely to respond?
- What do you think might be achieved?
- Do you think your response will empower your friend to share more?
- In what other way might you have responded?

Now take a look at a second possible interaction between you and your friend:

> Friend: '*I feel awful since they walked away, I feel so sad and empty. I am really worried.*'
>
> You: '*I am truly sorry to hear they left. You feel sad and you are worried? Can I ask what it is that is worrying you, do you feel it would help to talk about what you are feeling?*'

Now revisit the same questions above. Once you have answered the questions a second time, which would you consider to be the empathic response, whereby you are trying to convey to your friend that they can be heard and understood and just because you are their friend you are not going to assume to know?

Hopefully, you will have identified the second response as the empathic response. The first response, which is a sympathetic response, may convey a level of compassion to your friend but almost immediately it tells her that you don't understand her, and may even inhibit her from talking to you openly. I know myself when I have experienced the loss of a relationship, there are friends I can explore what I am going through with, because they listen to me, hear me, want to understand me, and there are friends who I would not wish to talk, just because they struggle not to tell me how I should be feeling and thinking.

Now what has this got to do with reflection? In order to reflect properly and gain the most from the process, we need to be able to understand ourselves, but that understanding needs to be accurate – understanding that is based upon not assuming to know how we think and feel about things. Such an understanding needs to come from an exploration of our true thoughts and feelings. Take a look at the example of reflection-on- action in Table 4.1. Here you will see an example of reflection where empathy is not available to the reflector and an example of where the person reflecting has embodied the notion of reflection and used empathic responding skills to get to know themselves with accuracy.

Table 4.1 Empathy in the reflective process – reflection-on-action

Without empathy	*The experience*	*With empathy*
I don't know why I didn't really listen to her. I think I just felt that having done some reading I knew best. I have learned that I need to listen more and demonstrate I have heard the person more clearly	I was supporting a lady in the community who was terrified of having a natural birth and was determined to move forward with a caesarean section. The lady was engaged with mental health services due to low mood, anxiety and post-natal depression following the birth of her first child. She had also had a very traumatic natural birth with her first child where mum and baby both nearly died. I strongly advised her to have a natural birth, advising that recovery from a caesarean section is prolonged and there can be complications. I did not support or listen to her when she was expressing her concerns about the natural birth; in fact, I was quite dismissive. As a result, I feel that I am now struggling to connect with her.	I didn't listen to her concerns with care and compassion. I have asked myself why. At first I believed it to be because I had done some reading around birthing methods and I felt I was being truly evidenced-based in my reaction. However, I have considered this more deeply and I recognize that I was bringing elements of myself into my interaction and it was clouding my judgement. Thinking about my own experiences of a caesarean section, I now recognize they were hindering my ability to truly hear her concerns. I have recognized here that my own experiences and feelings and thoughts about those experiences were not put to one side. This hindered my ability to be with this lady.

Before we revisit the extended description of reflection, take another look at the exercises in this chapter where you have provided your own understanding of the concepts we have discussed. Would you now change those definitions in light of what has been discussed?

By revisiting the extended description of reflection here, we can see where the ingredients of being person-centred and being empathic are situated:

> *'Reflection is an essential, engaging process that allows the reflector to frame and reframe their reality that is, and has been experienced moment by moment. Actively participating in the reflective process – that is, in, on or before an experience – requires us to tell our story and meander through that narrative, allowing ourselves to move where our thoughts and feelings wish to take us. It requires us to utilize skills of communication, to communicate with ourselves authentically, to become our own person-centred enquirer, understanding ourselves in relation to experiences we are about to have, are having or have had, empathically and with accuracy.'*

Key points that can be taken from this chapter are:

- Being person-centred plays a vital role in ensuring effective successful reflection.
- Being person-centred provides a framework that allows us to get to know our true selves.
- The core conditions of genuineness, unconditional positive regard and empathy are the cornerstones of being person-centred.
- You cannot truly be empathic without embodying the core conditions of genuineness and unconditional positive regard.
- In order to truly understand yourself, you have to assume not to know – and you need to want to get to know – yourself with accuracy.
- Empathy supports the accuracy of understanding in the reflective process.
- Being person-centred is a way of 'being', not just a skill set.

CHAPTER

5

Communication and mindfulness

Essential ingredient #7: Communication

The person reflecting needs to be able to articulate in a verbal and non-verbal manner, whether this is to themselves or to another person. They need to have the communication skills that allow them to act as their own internal supervisor. These communication skills include the skills of Socratic questioning and empathic responding in order to be able to investigate and enquire deeply into their experiences.

Essential ingredient #8: Mindfulness

The person reflecting needs to be present with themselves, aware of how their surroundings are and will guide their behaviours, thoughts and feelings within experiences. An acute awareness of how their values and belief systems, along with culture, policy and the political sphere will influence who they are in the context of others.

Learning outcomes

By the end of this chapter, you will be able to:

- Identify how and what communication skills support successful reflection.
- Use knowledge of Socratic dialogue and empathic responding to investigate your experiences deeply.
- Articulate the meaning of 'internal supervisor'.
- Practise using the basic skills of Socratic dialogue and empathic responding in the reflective process, whether with another person or when acting as your own internal supervisor.
- Use the knowledge of mindfulness to connect to yourself within your experiences.
- Use mindfulness to understand yourself in the context of others.
- Know the meaning of reflexivity.

In the previous chapter, we saw how important being *person-centred* and *empathic* are to the reflective process. We took a detailed look at these terms and their relationship with reflection. We discovered that being person-centred with ourselves when reflecting supports a deeper understanding of our true selves. It provides a framework that empowers us to be free and honest with our thoughts and feelings. We also established that the third core condition of the approach – empathy – is fundamental to empowering and enabling us to be person-centred. However, we also learned that empathy is not only about truly wanting to get to know ourselves from our own unique perspective but is also a set of communication skills. If we look at the following element of the extended description of reflection, we can see reference to a further dimension of person-centredness:

> '*It requires us to utilize skills of communication, to communicate with ourselves authentically, to become our own person-centred enquirer, understanding ourselves in relation to experiences we are about to have, are having or have had, empathically and with accuracy. Then stepping beyond the*

self and using this knowledge gained to understand how we may then have influenced those around us.'

This further dimension asks us to use the knowledge gained about ourselves in the reflective process from being person-centred and consider what we have learned in the context of others, how we may have influenced those around us. This requires us to be reflexive and mindful.

The aims of this chapter are twofold: first, to explore communication as it relates to the reflective process, identifying the skills of Socratic dialogue and empathic responding and how we can apply these skills to ourselves when reflecting; and second, to discuss mindfulness in the context of the reflective process and how it also relates to the notion of reflexivity.

Let us now take a look at our seventh essential ingredient – *communication*.

Communication

Essential ingredient #7: Communication

The person reflecting needs to be able to articulate in a verbal and non-verbal manner, whether this is to themselves or to another person. They need to have the communication skills that allow them to act as their own internal supervisor. These communication skills include the skills of Socratic questioning and empathic responding in order to be able to investigate and enquire deeply into their experiences.

Have a go at completing Exercises 5.1 and 5.2.

Exercise 5.1: Communication skills

From what you have read so far, jot down the communication skills and techniques you are aware of.

Exercise 5.2: Exploring your knowledge of communication in the reflective process

Having read the previous chapters and drawing on what you wrote for Exercise 5.1, jot down why you think communication is vital to the reflective process and which skills from Exercise 5.1 are most important.

We all communicate to one degree or another and we know we can communicate in different ways. The fact that we are referring here to communication skills implies that ways, methods and techniques of communicating are, over time, practised, developed and hopefully used with a purpose in mind. In healthcare, communication skills such as active listening and the use of both verbal and non-verbal cues are integral to the development of the therapeutic relationship with the person you are caring for or helping. Listening in healthcare not only allows you to gather accurate information, for if you listen actively – that is, concentrate on what the person is telling you, really trying to hear what they are saying, and relaying back to them that you understand – the service user will feel heard and understood, which ultimately helps to create an environment that may empower them to feel safe enough to talk to you. This process of actively listening is aided by your verbal and non-verbal skills. The use of these verbal and non-verbal skills will develop over time; the more you practise and reflect on your experiences of communicating, the more you will understand the way you communicate with others. What we wish to do here is develop these skills in relation to *yourself* in the reflective process.

This is not a simple task, as it is not every day you are asked to consider how you communicate with yourself. So, before we move on, ask yourself how often you talk to yourself. How often do you stop and have a conversation with yourself about what you are experiencing? I would suggest possibly not as often as you will do once you have finished reading this book and become proficient at being your own *internal supervisor*.

The internal supervisor

Earlier, we acknowledged the different times when reflection can occur. You may remember that we can reflect both 'on' and 'in' experience (see Figure 5.1). In the literature, historically, it is acknowledged that spontaneous reflection in-experience is not only a product of the development of reflecting on-experience skills but of the development of our internal supervisor (Casement, 1985; Bond and Holland, 1998; Todd, 2005). Let us consider what we mean by the idea of the internal supervisor.

On-experience Reflection occurs following the experience.	**In-experience** Reflection occurs in the moment of the experience, at the time – thinking on your feet!

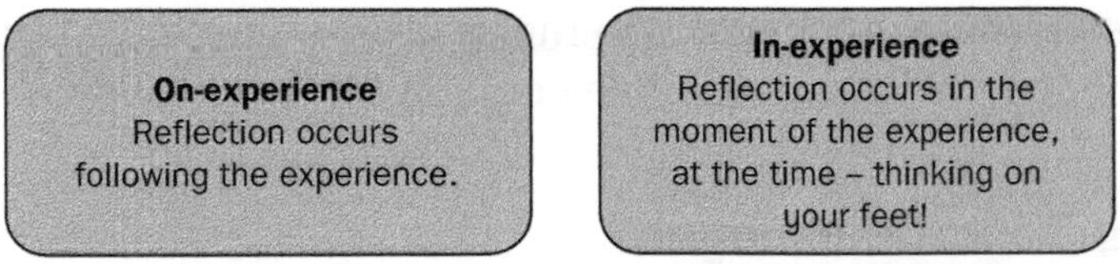

Figure 5.1 Reflection-on-experience and reflection-in-experience

The notion of the 'internal supervisor' was devised as a metaphor to describe the dialogue that occurs in our minds when we reflect after the moment of an experience, or the conversation that a person holds with him or herself internally about an experience as that experience is unfolding (Todd, 2005). The internal supervisor (you) will question personal bias (judgements) and subjectivity in the hope that you will find a more objective perspective and way of looking at something (Todd, 2002). The internal supervisor is a way of questioning the self or yourself at the time of engaging in a given situation – it allows you to be fully aware of your own engagement and to be mindful of the potential outcome. This is not easy to do and will take practice. Being able to question personal bias requires you to be open to challenging yourself, along with courage and honesty, qualities we discussed in the previous chapter.

The internal supervisor will listen and question more than it will talk but, in the questioning, it will use skills of communication that include Socratic dialogue and empathic questioning and responding, which we will address later in this chapter. By activating our internal supervisor, we are able to reflect in-experience, on-experience and pre-experience, and as a result become intentionally mindful. For example:

> '*I am feeling really insecure about what I am doing. I think my mentor is waiting for me to fail, she is constantly watching me.*'

> '*Waiting for me to fail? Do I really think this person wants me to fail, why am I thinking this, where has this come from. What is it that is happening to make me think this?*'

Johns (2000) has acknowledged that there are limits to reflecting alone, and that guided reflection with another person who can take over the role of internal supervisor can allow the reflective process to become more meaningful – this is something I discuss in detail in a later chapter. However, if we have no one to reflect with and we want to reflect in, after or before the moment, we need to understand the types of communication skills needed by our own internal supervisor. These skills relate to the two terms we have previously acknowledged: Socratic dialogue and empathic responding.

What is Socratic dialogue?

Socratic dialogue refers to systems devised by the Greek philosopher Socrates called 'Socratic methods'. In simple terms, Socratic dialogue aims to question our preconceived ideas and predetermined knowledge. Socratic questioning assumes 'not knowing' (i.e. have no knowledge about the subject in question) but by asking probing questions that require evidence for an answer, aims to achieve a deeper level of understanding about a particular topic. The aim of Socratic questioning and dialogue is to explore through 'guided discovery' the content and meaning of experiences to enable learning to take place, and thus allow for change to occur in cognition/thought and behaviour (Wells, 1997). This type of dialogue is a means of communication that allows for a deep analysis/exploration of self, through probing and gentle questioning. Although there may be no concrete answers, information is generated that enables us to become more deeply familiar with our own selves (Ciarrochi and Bailey, 2008).

Now have a go at Exercise 5.3.

Exercise 5.3: Types of questions for a Socratic dialogue with yourself

This exercise is about *you* recalling an experience you have had. Your recall may be based on having written this experience down, as in the example below, or you may have simply remembered it and be left with feelings that arose as part of the experience, or that arose following the experience.

Now, jot down any questions you would ask yourself to provide more information about the experience you have chosen. Remember that what you are trying to do here is probe more deeply and gain a better understanding of the experience. You don't want to make assumptions about yourself; instead, by being person-centred and using Socratic dialogue, you want to explore the things you say you feel, and think more deeply, to question, dispute or confirm your thoughts and feelings.

Example scenario:

'I really enjoyed placement today. I think that might be the first time that I felt comfortable and part of the team. I was able to apply finally what I have been learning in class. I don't think I have truly connected with the module yet, until today. It just seemed to click today. I was given responsibility today, maybe that's why, I am not sure why I have not been trusted enough to do anything by my myself yet. Maybe it's just me, maybe it is something I am doing, but I don't know what I did differently today.'

Thinking of questions to ask is not a simple task, especially when it is ourselves we are enquiring about, so I'm guessing that that wasn't the easiest of tasks for you. But as I stated earlier, the more you practise, the easier it will become.

Now let us take a look at a model of reflection that will provide a framework for you until you are proficient and comfortable holding a Socratic dialogue with yourself. Johns' model of structured reflection (one of my favourites as I find the questions really helpful) is composed of a series of questions that should help you when reflecting to focus in on a specific experience, and by using the questions highlighted in **bold** to hold a more Socratic dialogue with yourself (see Box 5.1). This model of reflection will likely be more useful if you are reflecting alone and are a novice reflector requiring a more structured format. Johns' model is aimed at helping us to gain an empathic understanding of self, in relation to the experience we have had. This model does not assume that we know the questions to ask of ourselves. It does, however, require us to act in a non-judgemental way and offer unconditional positive regard to ourselves while reflecting, otherwise the honesty that forms part of the basis of any effective reflection may be hindered or reduced.

Box 5.1: A model of structured reflection

Reflective cue:

- Bring the mind home – re-immerse yourself in the experience.
- **Focus on a description of an experience that seems significant in some way.**
- **What resonated with me most starkly, what particular issues seem significant enough to demand attention?**
- **How do I think others were feeling, and what do I think made them feel that way?**
- **How was I feeling and what made me feel that way?**
- **What was I trying to achieve, and how did I respond?**
- *What were the consequences of my actions on the patient, others, myself?*
- **What factors influenced the way I was feeling, thinking or responding?**
- What knowledge informed or might have informed me?
- **To what extent did I act for the best and in tune with my own values?**
- **How does this situation connect with previous experiences?**
- How might I respond more effectively if the same circumstances were to arise again?
- *What would be the consequences of alternative actions for the patient, others, myself?*
- **How do I feel NOW about this experience?**
- Am I more able to support myself and others as a consequence?
- Am I more able to realize desirable practice monitored using appropriate frameworks such as framing perspectives, Carper's fundamental ways of knowing or other maps?

Source: Adapted from Johns (2005: 3).

This model is also useful as it reminds us to consider ourselves in the context of others. As the reflector, you are asked to take into account the impact you may have had on those around you while in your experience. You need to remember we don't experience in isolation; any experience we have that has other people in it, in whatever guise, means these others will experience us, have our experience! The questions in *italics* in Box 5.1 require us to be reflexive and mindful, concepts that will be discussed later in the chapter. However, what this model doesn't do is give us the extra, probing questions and responses that push us to explore more deeply to uncover the layers of who we are and really understand ourselves accurately and allow us to feel heard by ourselves. The skills of empathic responding can help us with this.

This type of reflective conversation that we have with ourselves, engaging our internal supervisor in a conversation that includes the skills of Socratic dialogue and empathic responding, is of utmost importance. It is an interactive process that allows us to construct and reconstruct meaning and action related to our experiences, called *framing* and *reframing* by Schön (1983). If we perceive something we have experienced to be really awful and we believe ourselves to be totally at fault, reflecting using Socratic dialogue and empathic responding techniques will not only frame our experience but also allow us to potentially view our experience quite differently, which is reframing. Indeed, by reframing the experience, we might conclude we were not at fault. So, instead of ruminating and internalizing an incorrect interpretation of our experiences, the reflective process can help us to internalize the experience differently and more accurately. At the least, it will enable us to learn something about ourselves.

Let us now take a look at what we mean by empathic responding skills. Rogers (1980) was very clear when he suggested that true empathy is free of any judgement or analytical quality. Therefore, our responding skills need to be skills that probe our inner world and allow us to express accurately what we truly think and feel about our experiences. In the previous chapter, we explored the meaning of empathy. Let us now consider what the skills of empathy are.

Have a go at completing Exercise 5.4.

Exercise 5.4: Empathic responding skills

Jot down ways of responding to a person or yourself in an empathic manner. What types of communication skills do you know that would allow you to tell yourself in more detail what you think and feel, as well as allow you to check the accuracy of your understanding? What empathic responding skills might I use?

Now compare what you wrote down with the following:

- open questions;
- reflecting – parrot phrasing – mirroring;
- paraphrasing;
- exploring;
- clarifying;
- understanding ambivalence.

Did you record any of these empathic responding skills? None of these skills involves making interpretations, analysis or guesswork. They are all underpinned by the discussion on being person-centred we had in the previous chapter. Figure 5.2 details what each of the communication skills of empathic responding entails. Do you think you have used any of these in your training so far, or with another person in any situation? Ask yourself if there are any particular skills you need to practise.

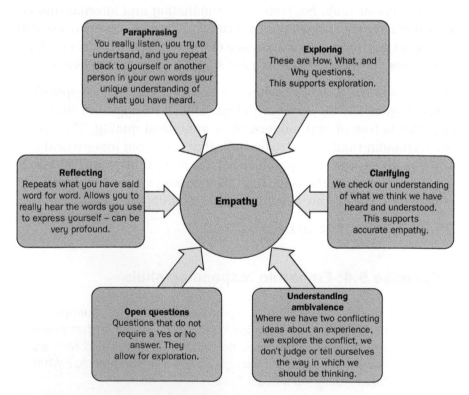

Figure 5.2 Empathic responding skills

Rogers (1980) advised us to remember that empathy is not just a skill set but also an attitude underpinned with genuine curiosity and unconditional positive regard towards the person – in this case, our-selves – who we are trying to understand. So, we can start to see how our ingredients interconnect.

A word or two is required about ambivalence. This is a term that is part of a counselling school of thought called 'motivational interviewing'. Having used motivational interviewing a lot with my service users who have a substance misuse disorder, I find it to be extremely useful in the person-centred helping relationship and as such you can apply it to yourself in the reflective process. Ambivalence is a common state that occurs when contradictory or incompatible emotions or attitudes co-exist in the same individual, and tension arises as a consequence (Miller and Rollnick, 2002). Asking questions about the ambivalence in order to understand it in the reflective process can also help you to resolve your ambivalence. Here are a couple of examples of incompatible thoughts.

> *'I really want to stop smoking. I hate the smell and the worry I have about my health, but I really enjoy smoking and the feel of the burn in the back of my throat …'*

> *'I really want help with my numeracy exam, but I don't want to ask as I feel stupid doing so …'*

Here we can see two different types of ambivalence. The first is a form of ambivalence typically displayed in my experience by people who smoke. The second is not untypical of my students who are concerned about what people will think of them if they ask for help. When asking ourselves questions, we may reveal ambivalences when conflicting ideas or thoughts arise, and further questions can help us to explore the conflict in thinking and may even provide answers to help resolve those ambivalences.

Before we look at our next essential ingredient, mindfulness, practise the skills of Socratic questioning and empathic responding when reflecting on yourself. Practise them on your friends, family and work colleagues; try and use them in general conversation. In this way, it is hoped it will become natural for you to embody what it means to be empathic and using it yourself when reflecting will become easier.

Let us now take a look at our eighth essential ingredient – *mindfulness*.

Mindfulness

Essential ingredient #8: Mindfulness

The person reflecting needs to be present with themselves, aware of how their surroundings are and will guide their behaviours, thoughts and feelings within experiences. An acute awareness of how their values and belief systems, along with culture, policy and the political sphere will influence who they are in the context of others.

It was acknowledged earlier in this chapter that the extended description of reflection asks us to use the knowledge gained about ourselves from being person-centred in the reflective process and to consider what we have learned about ourselves in the context of others. Now that we also have the communication skills required to get to know ourselves accurately, we can take this a step further and become *reflexive* and *mindful*. Mindfulness in this context means being connected to ourselves, fully present with who we are and aware of ourselves moment to moment, but also aware of who we are in the context of others – that is, how are we affecting those around us and how they are influencing us. So, let us consider what being mindful means and how it can relate to being reflexive.

Have a look at the following experience, which is based on my memory of giving my first injection.

> *'I remember being in the second year of my four-year degree in mental health nursing. I had been given an adult branch placement in the hospital general setting. My mentor was supervising me give my very first injection. This, I recall, was a heparin injection. In my mind's eye, I can remember the needle being and feeling huge with a great big scoop on the end. It looked blunt to me, although I know it wasn't. I can recall thinking that it will be me that puts it in the wrong place and damages the patient. I remember the older patient's tummy being very wrinkly and leathery. I remember watching almost in slow motion as my hand darted the needle towards the skin and then it bounced off! I remember my heart being in my mouth, I*

remember sweating in my very starchy, blue, unforgiving uniform, shaking, and so hoping that my mentor would take over from me, which she did not do. She made me do it again. The second time I managed to complete the procedure successfully. I recall an immediate sense of relief, feeling very proud of my young self, and hoping never to give another injection again!'

Back then, when I was 19 years old, I remember my reflections focused mostly on me rather than anything else. I reflected diligently on how I felt, and why I felt the way I did; I explored my thinking, I reflected conscientiously on how the procedure was influenced by my thinking and my feelings of anxiety. I challenged my thinking that I was always going to be that nurse who got it horribly wrong, I even read lots on giving injections and managing anxiety. I considered what I had learned from the experience. But now when I look back and remember, not once did I explore how my experience might have affected the person I was caring for. Not once did I consider how he might have experienced me. Because he did *experience* me.

I did reflect on how I felt about hurting him, but I did not reflect on how my nervousness and anxiety around hurting him impacted upon him. I did not consider how my thoughts, feelings and behaviour might have affected my mentor, who was attempting to teach me. So, although as a novice reflector I reflected quite well to a point, and I did learn things about me, it was in isolation from others and it was, to a degree, self-indulgent rumination. So being mindful helps to prevent what Bolton (2010) termed self-indulgent rumination.

What is meant by mindfulness in the context of reflection? According to Johns, a prominent writer in the field of reflection and nursing, reflective, mindful practice is framed as a 'way of being: a way that honours the intuitive and holistic nature of experience' (2005: 7). Note how this is not too dissimilar to the notion of being person-centred and embodying this notion as a *way of being*. Viewing reflection as being in a relationship with yourself and connected with the notion of mindfulness allows us to understand reflection as something that can not only be premeditated but be spontaneous, in the moment, at the time. It allows us to personify the notion of reflection and to reflect moment-by-moment, not just 'in' or 'on' experience. Johns (2005) further suggested that mindfulness is not only the thoughtful exclusion of everything except that which is being attended to, when attached to reflection it provides a framework within which we can view ourselves as a moment unfolds. But when being mindful, we don't just sit back and watch things happening to us. It is not a passive process. Instead, mindfulness in the reflective process means we are truly engaged with the unfolding situation and embodying all aspects of reflection so that we can understand ourselves at the time.

Bolton (2010) suggested mindfulness means that you are fully conscious of your actions, which in turn enables awareness of the likely outcome and appropriateness of the actions to be taken. Think about this in relation to driving. Some people drive on auto pilot. They perceive they know the car they drive and the road to where they need to go so well, that they stop thinking about it. They just drive and miraculously arrive where they need to be. This does not make for good driving, and this takes us back to what Schön (1983) called knowing-in-action, or only using technical rationality. A driver who is mindful drives with funnel vision, is aware of the ever-changing conditions of the road, is able to move with the rhythms of other cars on the road, will manoeuvre the car in accordance with the road conditions, and will be constantly aware of what is in their line of sight but also what their blind spots are. A mindful driver, in my opinion, makes for a better driver than the one who drives on auto pilot.

Let us consider this in relation to reflection pre-action. When adopting mindfulness, you don't just blunder into a situation unprepared, but contemplate, cogitate and reflect upon the potentiality of what is about to be encountered – though this could simply be classed as conscientious healthcare practice. As a student or as a qualified practitioner, before you embark on a new course of action (maybe you are giving a medication you have not given before, or meeting someone new), you should always diligently think about and explore what you are about to do. You may know that you already do this, so all we are doing here is giving a name to something you ensure happens and taking it a step further by ensuring you connect with who you are, not just the mechanics of the potential experience.

Mindfulness is a way of moving to a more purposeful way of perceiving experiences from a range of viewpoints and potential scenarios. Bolton (2010) likens the mindfulness in reflection to a game of chess in which a player (the reflector) does not make a move without considering first its impact on the rest of their own and their opponent's pieces, and what it might mean for the game as a whole (the experience). Thus, the player considers moving the piece not in isolation, but in among all the other chess pieces (life, work and people) and how their next move will impact upon the outcome of the game. This leads us effectively to the notion of reflexivity.

Reflexivity as an independent notion has been discussed and analysed in some detail in the literature (Archer, 2007; Bolton, 2010). As it relates to reflection and the reflective process, it simply means we wish to understand how others perceive us and how our external environment affects us. Reflexivity means finding strategies to question and challenge our attitudes, values, beliefs, ideas and behaviours to generate understanding of how these inform our role and the complexity of how our role interrelates with others. How does our behaviour and personal value set fit with organizational structure and context? How congruent are we in our behaviours in relation to the values and theories we embrace? (Bager-Charleson, 2010).

Let's return to my memory of my first injection. If I had been reflexive within the reflective process, I would have connected to myself not only after the moment but also in that moment. I would have tried to explore how the patient was feeling and had experienced me, how my values of being kind to another and my student nurse's code of conduct was influencing my behaviour. I was so terrified of hurting this person when I gave the injection it was really conflicting with my value set and inhibiting my behaviour.

This would have given me a different perspective, an added dimension – another way of viewing what happened. This would have resulted in a greater level of knowledge about myself that I could then have taken on board. Bolton (2010), in the creation of *through the mirror writing*, shows us how, through reflective writing, we can develop the ability to view our experiences from another person's perspective.

Have a go at Exercise 5.5.

Exercise 5.5: Being reflexive

First, write down your reflections on a recent experience you had that impacted upon you. Then, rewrite the experience from the point of view of another person who was part of your experience.

Now consider what learning has taken place, having analysed the experience from not only your own perspective but also that of another.

Can you see how reflecting upon your experience from another person's perspective will offer a different dimension to your learning? By being reflexive in the reflective process we are:

> … finding strategies to question our own attitudes, thought processes, values, assumptions, prejudices and habitual actions, to strive to understand our complex role in relation to others.
>
> (Bolton 2010:13)

Gaining that vital self-awareness in relation to how others perceive and experience us ensures not only a deeper level of reflection, especially when being mindful, but gives an added breadth of analysis. In essence, by being mindful in the reflective process, we are embodying the notion of reflection moment by moment. We are allowing it to become a more fluid, a less mechanical process that ensures we are aware of ourselves at the time we are having or are about to have our experiences. The added element of reflexivity ensures that our reflection is more than one-dimensional, in that we not only get to know ourselves, but also get to try and understand how we are influenced by values and bias, how our professional structures influence our behaviours and, of course, how other people view us.

By revisiting the extended description of reflection here, we can see where the ingredients of communication and mindfulness are situated:

> '*Reflection is an essential, engaging process that allows the reflector to frame and reframe their reality that is, and has been experienced moment by moment. Actively participating in the reflective process – that is, in, on or before an experience – requires us to tell our story and meander through that narrative, allowing ourselves to move where our thoughts and feelings wish to take us. It requires us to utilize skills of communication, to communicate with ourselves authentically, to become our own person-centred enquirer, understanding ourselves in relation to experiences we are about to have, are having or have had, empathically and with accuracy. Then stepping beyond the self and using this knowledge gained to understand how we may then have influenced those around us. To be fully immersed in this process, we must be open to learning about what constitutes 'I', leaving arrogance and*

complacency at the door, be kind and compassionate enough to offer ourselves unconditional positive regard, be actively engaged in mindfulness, and consciously aware of the self in our moments. Through a critical, analytical lens, we need to explore our experiences within the frame of how our history/ background and current locus, culture and context influence who we are in our moments. Reflection requires us to open ourselves up to sourcing and learning new knowledge if the knowledge is not already known to us.'

Key points that can be taken from this chapter are:

- When reflecting alone we need to become our own internal supervisor.
- Communication skills play a vital role in supporting us to get to know ourselves within the reflective process.
- The use of Socratic dialogue helps us to ensure that the questioning we apply to get to know ourselves allows for honesty and a deeper level of learning.
- Empathic responding skills are supported by the empathic attitude discussed in Chapter 1.
- Empathic responding skills ensure we probe more deeply when we get to know ourselves and that we are accurate in our understanding of self.
- Being mindful ensures that reflection is not a mechanical process.
- Being mindful allows us to be acutely aware of, and connected to, ourselves moment to moment.
- The reflexivity involved in the reflective process allows us to understand that we are not only affected by our own thoughts and feelings, but also by the context within which we have our experiences, understanding ourselves from another person's perspective, ensuring reflection is multidimensional.

Being process-orientated and being deliberate

Essential ingredient #9: Being process-orientated

Reflection is not about the outcome/output, but about the process that takes place when reflecting. Reflection may not always be so smooth as to guarantee a definitive outcome. When entering the reflective process, the person reflecting needs to meander and follow their own flow of feeling or train of thought. As much learning can take place from the process as can occur from the result.

Essential ingredient #10: Being deliberate

Reflecting is not a flippant, inconsequential recap of an event, but a deliberate, controlled, conscious, exploratory consideration of an experience. It is not just thinking! Engaging in the reflective process gives the reflector permission to take purposeful time to stop and spend moments with themselves. The reflector must also be cognisant that every decision they make as a result of reflection has a 'ripple effect'. The actions they take from the reflective process will not only impact upon the person reflecting but on those around them.

Learning outcomes

By the end of this chapter, you will be able to:

- Recognize how reflection is process-orientated.
- Acknowledge that learning can take place during the process of reflecting.
- Recognize that reflection is a deliberate and considered process.
- Understand that the decisions we put into practice as a result of reflecting will affect those around us and other areas of our lives.

In the previous chapters, we have explored in detail eight of the ten essential ingredients for successful reflection. By introducing you to and examining these eight essential ingredients in detail, I hope you have learned how reflection is so much more than just evaluating what we have done well and what we have done not so well. We have come to realize that reflection is an analysis of ourselves, our thoughts, feelings and behaviours, through and within the experiences we are going to have, have had or are having. We have discovered that we wish to *know* ourselves and so we want to reflect. To have self-awareness is to be able to really understand 'me', to highlight and fill any gaps in our ever-expanding knowledge of self and ultimately to enhance our levels of emotional intelligence in relation to knowing 'me', knowing how 'me' influences others, how 'me' is influenced by everything around us and how to use 'me' in the helping relationship.

We have established that the eight ingredients we have discussed so far support our ability to reflect. We have found that critical thinking skills underpin our ability to explore our experiences analytically, and to question what we do, see, feel and think. We have learned not to take anything at face value but to investigate and explore. These skills allow us to recognize also what our current knowledge is, and then use this to discover new knowledge.

We now know that our attitude – the bravery and courage we possess – is important in motivating us to want to get to know ourselves and support the honesty required of us to be our authentic selves in the reflective process. That our wanting to truly understand ourselves accurately, situating ourselves within a person-centred framework when reflecting, helps our empathy to be accurate, allowing for greater knowledge of self and therefore self-understanding. And finally, we have learned that the whole reflective process cannot operate unless we communicate both with ourselves and with others who offer us guided reflection, something we will explore in depth in a later chapter.

In this chapter, we will examine our final two essential ingredients before addressing how to put all of what we have learned together as a package (like baking a cake), in order to engage in the reflective process both verbally and in written form. It is the purpose of this chapter to address the notions of *process* and *being deliberate*. We will focus here on understanding how the learning that occurs because of reflection doesn't simply materialize at the end of the process, but that we are able to learn throughout the whole process. We will see that through the process of reflection, by putting all of the ingredients into the mix, pervasive learning can occur. We will also see that reflection, and what we do with what we learn, needs to be deliberate in order for it to become reflective practice.

Bolton sees reflection as a 'state of mind, an on-going constituent of practice, not a technique or curriculum element' (2010: 3). In other words, it is a way of 'being', an embodiment of thinking and behaving in a particular way; reflection can permeate who we are and it is a process that constantly encourages learning and the generation of emotional intelligence.

So, with this in mind, let us take a look at our ninth essential ingredient – *being process-orientated*.

Being process-orientated

Essential ingredient #9: Being process-orientated

Reflection is not about the outcome/output, but about the process that takes place when reflecting. Reflection may not always be so smooth as to guarantee a definitive outcome. When entering the reflective process, the person reflecting needs to meander and follow their own flow of feeling or train of thought. As much learning can take place from the process as can occur from the result.

First, have a go at completing Exercise 6.1.

Exercise 6.1: Defining process

Jot down what you think the word 'process' means, then what we mean when using 'process' in the context of reflection.

In thinking about the word 'process', I expect that you may have suggested the steps taken to achieve a particular outcome, or the things we do to achieve a particular result. Those of you who have come across reflection as part of your programme of study may have suggested that process in relation to reflection is to *describe* the experience, consider your *thoughts and feelings,* to *evaluate and analyse* this experience, and then decide on further *action* to be taken. The portrayal of process in this rigid, segregated manner (which is often as a result of being taught reflective models without being taught the underpinning philosophy of reflection itself) lacks the breadth and depth of understanding that we now know is the reflective process.

Let us review for a moment what we have learned so far about reflection in the previous chapters. Previous chapters have taught us that, process as it relates to reflection is about engaging in enquiry into self; the deep contemplation and exploration of what we truly think and feel; the act of pondering and investigating these thoughts and feelings and examining these in the context of our experiences; the attentive connection to self and consideration of our behaviour; the recognition of our current knowledge; the seeking out of new knowledge; the act of getting to know ourselves; and the thoughtfulness and mindfulness that is required if we are to consider those around us and how they experience us. These are aspects that are moved fluidly through. But also, aspects that we can reverse, move forward again, go sideways and ultimately meander through within the process of what we know as reflection. Take another look at the reflective process in Figure 6.1.

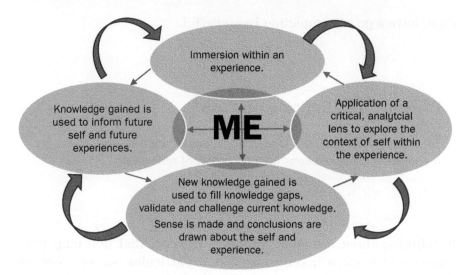

Figure 6.1 The reflective process

To show how learning can take place through the process of engaging in an experience and not just as the result of the experience, which demonstrates how we can learn in the process of reflecting not just from the result, let us look at a few real-life examples. The first two are normal activities that many people will participate in at some point in their lives, while the third is an activity engaged in by the majority of students on most courses.

In the first example, the outcome is a cake (Figure 6.2). When you ate the cake, which is the outcome – or the result of reflection – you almost certainly will have considered its consistency, its taste, even the way it looks. You will have learned also from the outcome, which is the cake, what is aesthetically pleasing to you and what your taste buds respond to. What we are concerned with here though, is to show that we can learn from the *process* of baking the cake – that is, the process of reflecting – as well from the end result, what the cake when baked tells us.

Take a look at Figure 6.2 and imagine that this is your first attempt at baking a cake. You will see some of the learning that will have occurred during the process of baking. By the time the cake has been baked, you will have learned about ingredients, measurements, conversions, timings and how to use an appliance. You will have learned also about yourself. Did you enjoy baking? Did you have a sense of achievement? Satisfaction? You will have considered and contemplated combinations of flavours, getting to know what you like and don't like. You will have recognized gaps in your knowledge, and you may have sought new knowledge to fill those gaps in order to bake the cake.

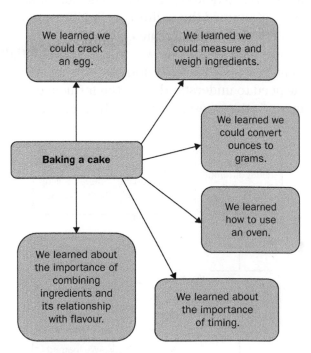

Figure 6.2 Learning from the process – baking your first cake

Our second example, which many of you will be able to identify with, is learning to drive a car. The outcome, or the result, is being able to drive. But in the process of learning to drive a car, we will have learned basic mechanical information – maybe also electronic information dependent upon the type of car – will have sourced new information to learn code, in this instance the highway code so we can recognize signage, road markings, etc., and read information in the car manual, so that we understand the car. We will have learned what our car can and cannot do in different gears, how weather influences how we handle the car, how others drive – we might even come to realize that others are not so good at driving, which might influence how we then drive. We will have learned that how we drive influences how others drive, and that our driving can have an effect on our passengers – if we are heavy on the break, jerky on the gears, we might make someone car-sick. In the process of learning to drive a car, we will have learned a multitude of other things too.

Now let's look at our third example, our first attempt at critically appraising a research article (Figure 6.3). The outcome, or the result, is that we have determined the validity, reliability and generalizability of the research and therefore the credibility of the findings. But within the process of appraisal, we will have potentially learned about different research methodologies, how to create research questions, the need to understand bias, the influence of sample size, the importance of ethics, researcher involvement, and so on.

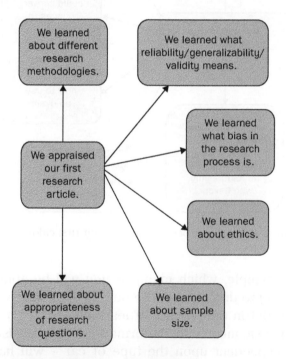

Figure 6.3 Appraising our first research article

These are just a few things we will have learned during the process of baking a cake, driving a car and appraising research. Although not exhaustive, they give us an idea of what can be learned in the process of having experiences as well as what can be learned from the outcome. As part of the process, you will have gained self-awareness and new knowledge – both theoretical and personal. So engaging in reflection is as much about the learning that can occur by moving through the process as it is about the outcome.

Learning taken from the process of reflection is not just an accumulation of facts; rather, it is the kind of learning that makes a difference to your behaviour, the course of action you might choose to take in the future, your attitudes and your personality. Carl Rogers, who we encountered in earlier chapters, refers to this type of learning as 'pervasive learning' – learning that is not just an accumulation of knowledge, but knowledge that interpenetrates every part of our existence (Rogers, 1967). When Rogers wrote about learning that can take place in the helping relationship, and more specifically within psychotherapy, he advised that there were several key areas for gaining knowledge. I have listed the ones here I believe to be most relevant to us today when receiving the learning that can occur from reflection:

- The person sees themselves differently in light of new knowledge.
- They accept themselves and their feelings more fully.
- They become more self-confident and self-directing.
- They become more the person they know themselves to be.
- They become more flexible, less rigid in their perceptions.
- They adopt more realistic goals for themselves.
- They behave in a more mature fashion.
- They change behaviours they perceive do not work for them.
- They become more accepting/understanding of others.
- They become more open to the evidence, both to what is going on outside themselves and what is going on inside themselves.
- They change in basic personality characteristics, in constructive ways.

For those of you who remain to be convinced about the learning that can take place, even having read the previous chapters, let us take a closer look at how these key areas and the reflective process are intertwined (Table 6.1).

Table 6.1 The key areas of pervasive learning and their relationship with the reflective process

Key area	Description
The person sees themselves differently in light of new knowledge	Reflection allows us to frame and reframe our experiences, it allows us to see those experiences from a different perspective and can provide us with new meanings. Being mindful and reflexive ensures we try and view how others perceive us in our experience and how we may influence them. We learn to know that we are influenced by our external environment and the contextual nature of that environment. As a result, we understand our experience from several different angles, which may allow us to see ourselves differently from first envisaged.
They accept themselves and their feelings more fully	The process of reflection teaches us that to be honest with ourselves about how we think and feel, to be empathic, we need to be non-judgemental. To really understand ourselves, we adopt a non-judgemental stance that enables true acceptance of what we would describe as 'me' or 'I'. We give ourselves permission to have that authentic voice.
They become more self-confident and self-directing	The process of reflecting allows us to practise honesty. This honesty supports the revealing of what we do and don't know. The act of engaging with what we don't know allows us to take action and to fill those gaps in our knowledge. We ultimately become more practised and therefore more comfortable with our ability to know what we do and don't know, and to source new knowledge. Increased capability increases self-confidence.
They become more the person they know themselves to be	The process of reflection wants us to use our current self-awareness to get to know ourselves more deeply, generating deeper levels of self-awareness. This process means that we can recognize what we know works for us and perhaps what doesn't, and as a result of the process we can make transformative changes to be more of the person we ultimately see and know ourselves to be.
They become more flexible, less rigid in their perceptions	The process of reflection, learning to be reflexive and mindful, helps us to realize that there is more than one view of a situation. In knowing that there is more than one way to perceive an experience and by knowing how others see us and what our impact is on them, we can learn to freely acknowledge and accept other perceptions and thus choose to be less rigid.

(continued)

Table 6.1 (Continued)

Key area	Description
They adopt more realistic goals for themselves	Engaging in the process of reflection persuades us to analyse and explore our experiences. If we do this openly and honestly, we can view our experiences and the realness of them. We can determine if the expectations we have of ourselves are reasonable. Through analysis and investigation, we can alter and adapt our expectations and goals. This part of the process helps us to not have unrealistic views of life as well as allowing us to expand our horizons if our goals and views are too narrow.
They behave in a more mature fashion	The process of reflection is about learning, not just about the mechanics of nursing or healthcare interventions, or lesson planning, but about ourselves. In the process of learning we become more emotionally mature, which leads to a greater emotional intelligence. This emotional intelligence can support not only professional practice, where we have greater understanding of how we are in the therapeutic relationship, but also in our personal lives, in the relationships we have with ourselves and family and friends. We can therefore behave and experience life in a more controlled, understood and mature way.
They change behaviours they perceive do not work for them	The insight we gain into ourselves from the process of reflection ensures we can understand our behaviour and why we think and feel the way we do. This understanding also means we get to know how we influence those around us. In essence, we get to know what works for us and what doesn't work. The more mature we become because of the process gives us the confidence to really acknowledge what works and allows us to change the behaviour, thoughts and feelings that are less useful to us.
They become more accepting/ understanding of others	In developing our ability to view our experiences from many different perspectives, we are able to see multiple realities. That our reality is just that, our reality, and others can experience our reality quite differently. The process teaches us to accept the different perspectives and to learn from this. As a result, we can choose to become more accepting of others because we learn that in our acceptance, we don't always need to agree.

(*continued*)

Table 6.1 (Continued)

Key area	Description
They become more open to the evidence, both to what is going on outside themselves and what is going on inside themselves	The process of reflection is all about understanding what is going on within ourselves and how we are impacted upon by our external environment. But the process of reflection teaches us to not just understand, but to be open to sourcing new knowledge. The process allows us to recognize the gaps we have in our knowledge and to be open to the evidence that could possibly fill those gaps.
They change in basic personality characteristics, in constructive ways	We know from previous chapters about the transformative nature of change that can occur within the reflective process. Through the process of reflection, we can learn about ourselves if we truly engage. If we truly engage and are open to the learning, we can change parts of who we are should we wish to do so. This change is not always conscious but the process can lead to subtle change that allows us to be the *best version of ourselves*.

Source: Rogers (1967).

We can see here the absolute potential for the pervasive learning that Rogers' key areas can foster in the process of reflection. Ultimately, these key areas relate to a learning about ourselves that allows us to become the person we want to be, it allows us to truly understand ourselves so we can adjust our behaviours if we need to. This type of learning allows us to achieve a level of emotional intelligence that facilitates understanding of the relationship we have with our external environment, and an understanding of those around us in a way that supports our recognition and acceptance of our influence on others. This pervasive learning is the knowledge and wisdom we are endeavouring to achieve through the process of reflecting for ourselves. As a trainee nurse, healthcare practitioner or educator, you will endeavour to impart this to your service users, the people you are helping, supporting them so that their own learning can help them to live their lives to their own unique potential.

Exercise 6.2: The key areas of pervasive learning

Take a look at the key areas of pervasive learning again. What do you think of the descriptions I have provided of the relationship each area has with the process of reflection? Are there any other areas that you would like to add?

Adding to our discussion on process and learning, Dalley (2009) recognized that the process of reflection can be as important as the outcome depending on the context within which we are reflecting. Dalley believed that the purpose of reflection is also about the acquisition of skills and learning during the actual process:

> Whether the purpose is seeking the outcomes of reflection or seeking the development of reflective skills *per se*. Is the outcome considered more important? Or is the process by which that outcome is arrived at considered the more important?
>
> (Dalley 2009: 19)

Consider the following two examples. The first is that of a nurse who perceives himself to be reflecting on why a patient of his is not responding to their prescribed dose of insulin. The nurse may not place much importance on the process of reflection; he may be more interested in the answer to his question, which is the 'outcome'.

The second is that of a nurse who perceives herself to be reflecting on why she responded to and felt a certain way about a particular patient. To this nurse, the process of reflection – getting to know herself, being mindful, reflexive, processing thoughts and feelings in the reflective process, going through Rogers' key areas – may be just as important, if not more so, than answering a question that may or may not have a definitive outcome.

We can see here two purposes perceived as reflection: the first is outcome-driven, the second process-driven. The first nurse may perceive that learning only takes place when reflecting to produce an outcome to an event, which as we know, is less reflection and more evaluation of practice. This is very different to the second nurse, who is trying to understand herself through the process of reflecting. Neither is incorrect, since it is important to evaluate practice and it is important to reflect. But what we need to understand is that if we engage in the process of reflecting rather than just focusing on the outcome of evaluating, far more learning about self can take place. And although there might not always be a definitive outcome as a result of reflection, there will always be a process that learning can occur within.

So let's give it a try. Have a look at Exercise 6.3.

Exercise 6.3: Learning from the process

First, consider an experience that had a marked impact on you. Maybe an experience you have had as part of your programme of study, or an experience you had outside university. Then, using the framework below, provide a brief description of the experience before breaking that experience down into sections or stages, as in Figures 6.2 and 6.3. Consider each section in turn and write down the learning you took from it (this is the process).

Brief description of the experience	Process sections	Learning taken from each section	Learning as a result of the overall outcome

Next, consider the experience as a whole and jot down the overall learning taken from the experience (this is the outcome). While undertaking this exercise, bear in mind the other essential ingredients for successful reflection and underpin this with Rogers' key areas of pervasive learning. Put those ingredients into action when undertaking this exercise.

What you are doing here is teaching yourself how to reflect – putting all the previous ingredients into practice to show how reflection is a process and how learning can be taken from this process. You should learn as much from breaking down the experience and reflecting on the process of the experience as you do from reflecting on the outcome. This breaking down of a topic into its component parts and exploring the meaning, through investigation and analysis, is also critical thinking in action.

If we revisit the extended description of reflection, we can see where this ingredient is situated:

> 'Reflection is an essential, engaging process that allows the reflector to frame and reframe their reality that is, and has been experienced moment by moment. Actively participating

in the reflective process – that is, in, on or before an experi-
ence – requires us to tell our story and meander through that
narrative, allowing ourselves to move where our thoughts and
feelings wish to take us.'

Let's now take a look at our tenth and final essential ingredient for successful reflection – *being deliberate.*

Being deliberate

Essential ingredient #10: Being deliberate

Reflecting is not a flippant, inconsequential recap of an event, but a delib-
erate, controlled, conscious, exploratory consideration of an experience.
It is not just thinking! Engaging in the reflective process gives the reflector
permission to take purposeful time to stop and spend moments with
themselves. The reflector must also be cognisant that every decision they
make as a result of reflection has a 'ripple effect'. The actions they take
from the reflective process will not only impact upon the person reflecting
but on those around them.

You will notice that I have altered the name of this ingredient from *strategic* to *deliberate*. Again, this is a result of having reviewed my previous research and thoughts in light of my own developed thinking. For me the word 'deliberate' embraces the notions of consciously, intentionally, carefully and unhurried – considered. This for me is how we reflect. On reflection, the word strategic for me implies a more business-like focus, with slightly less humanness to it; I think of military planning rather than mindfully engaging in reflection and as we know reflection is highly human. As a result, I have changed the name of this ingredient.

This ingredient is therefore about recognizing that reflection is *deliberate* – that it is not an ad hoc recollection of events, or a brief flippant consideration of how we are behaving. Reflection is very meaningful and involves deliberate, thoughtful consideration of our experiences. Even reflecting in the moment, where we are mindful, is a conscious, intentional consideration of who we are, what we are, how we are. During your training, you have likely been introduced to reflective models and cycles, which provide a framework within which to reflect. These models (for example, those of Borton, Gibbs, Atkins and Murphy) recognize the deliberate, considered nature of reflection and the importance of ensuring the reflector is supported during the process. However, as I noted earlier, these models will only be used correctly if the underpinning philosophy of reflection is understood.

In Chapter 7, I introduce my own reflective framework: the EESI framework, where EESI = 'Experience, Exploration, Sense-making, Implementation'.

Technical reflection

In addition to reflective models, writers on reflection have also alluded to the deliberate nature of reflection. When discussing reflection in relation to clinical practice and formulating evaluation of practice as reflection, Taylor (2000) referred to the notion of *technical reflection*, which she perceives as a level of reflection that requires nurses to think critically and reason scientifically about what they have learned in the reflective process so that they can critique and adjust current behaviours/ways of working when necessary. Technical reflection is deliberate and is about influencing clinical practice. This type of reflection is outcome-driven and more akin to critical incident analysis whereby we deliberately consider the mechanics of interventions in the clinical area and relate our learning to the current evidence base. However, technical reflection is still underpinned by the information we have discussed in previous chapters, in particular the ingredients of critical analysis and knowledge.

As you are now aware, even critical analysis is deliberate in its conscious and thoughtful exploration of experience in light of the evidence. So, Taylor (2000), having been influenced by authors such as Bandman and Bandman (1995) and Van Hooft et al. (1995), referred to technical reflection as the scientific reasoning and function of a critical thinker underpinned by the problem-solving steps of the nursing process, or any other process that has an evidence base (Wilkinson, 1996). Implementing the process of technical reflection involves developing an argument by analysing the issues and assumptions, managing the situation, planning and assessing, and evaluating the problem in light of all the information gained through the process of technical reflection. Overall, this is not at all dissimilar to the reflective process we have been discussing so far in this book, but with more focus potentially on the outcome. As a result, if we engage in Taylor's idea of technical reflection, the process will be undertaken in a thoughtful, considered and deliberate manner. Technical reflection highlights the deliberate process undertaken to ensure learning takes place when reflecting.

In writing about reflection, Van Manen (1995) broke the process down into four elements, demonstrating how deliberate reflection can be. Table 6.2 provides a commentary on each of these four elements. We can clearly see there are four very separate stages that are mindfully engaged with during the reflective process, further supporting the first part of the essential ingredient that is being deliberate:

> *'Reflecting is not a flippant, inconsequential recap of an event, but a deliberate, controlled, conscious, exploratory consideration of an experience. It is not just thinking!'*

We can also see how these stages align very closely with all the other ingredients in previous chapters. Table 6.2 highlights the very purposeful nature of reflection that Van Manen is alluding to, and the requirement to be very deliberate in that process.

Table 6.2 The four elements of reflection

Element	*Description*
Anticipatory	Before engaging in a task, the reflector is required to think about possible actions, interventions and likely outcomes, often referred to as pre-reflection.
Active	The reflector is able to maintain and promote awareness of what they are doing at any given time. This requires the reflector to be conscious of what they are doing at the time they are doing it.
Mindful	The reflector has developed and is developing the capacity to be actively reflective and thoughtful during the experiences that they are encountering, sometimes referred to as 'thinking on the job' or reflecting on-action.
Recollective	Having thought about the experience to be encountered, the reflector becomes consciously aware during the experience, reflects at the time of the experience, and is able to consider and evaluate the experience by addressing the success of any outcome.

Source: Adapted from Van Manen (1995).

Let us take a look now at the second part of the ingredient that is being deliberate.

> *'The reflector must also be cognisant that every decision they make as a result of reflection has a 'ripple effect'. The actions they take from the reflective process will not only impact upon the person reflecting but on those around them.'*

This second part requires us not only to recognize that reflection is a deliberate process, even when there isn't an outcome, but that our action based on the learning gained in the reflective process has a wider audience beyond ourselves.

In Chapter 5, where we addressed mindfulness, we learned that in the reflective process we must consider the influence our experiences have on those around us. We learned that reflection is more than just self-indulgent rumination – that learning about ourselves can be enhanced if we consider the influence our behaviour (including our thoughts and feelings) has on others. Being deliberate requires us to take this a step further. In being deliberate in the process, we need to consider the impact on others of any action we undertake or decision we make as a result of the reflective process – we need to be forward-thinking. That means reflecting not just on how we affect people during our experiences but also the effect we can have on them following the experience and reflection. This ingredient, therefore, requires us to think deliberately/purposefully about what we do with the learning before we take any kind of action; that is, consider the likely impact – both on ourselves and others – of our actions and future behaviours.

Exercise 6.4: Decision-making and the ripple effect

Can you recall a time when you made a decision to change your approach? Do you remember applying thoughtful consideration to the implications your approach might have had on your environment and those around you? Did you consider the 'ripple effect' or the knock-on effect your approach might have had?

To understand this notion of the ripple effect, let's take a look at something you might come across as a senior nurse or ward manager.

Scenario 6.1

You have reflected diligently and from the learning that has taken place you have decided to implement a change in practice on your ward. You decide to send all the ward staff on a three-day drug and alcohol training programme that occurs once a year, at a cost of £1,000 per person. Figure 6.4 highlights the potential impact of sending all the staff on this training course. Can you think of any other ways in which this training could have a wider impact, or create a ripple effect?

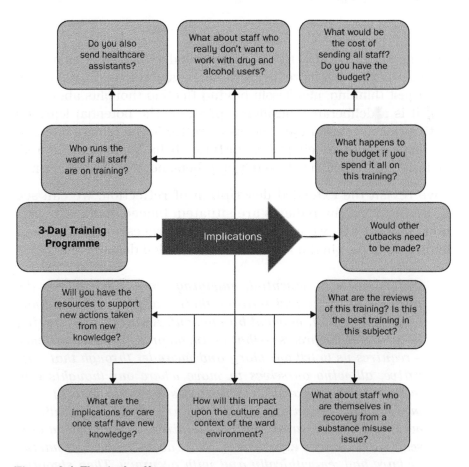

Figure 6.4 The ripple effect

A reflective manager would consider and analyse in the reflective process the impact this course of action might have before it is implemented. If the ripple effect were to result in some negative outcome, the course of action ought to be adapted.

Have a go at Exercise 6.5 – your own ripple effect.

Exercise 6.5: Your own ripple effect

Think of an occasion when you made a decision to alter or implement future actions or behaviours. Who and what else were you aware of being affected by the changes and implementations? What was the ripple effect, what were the implications?

This chapter has taught us that having understood reflection, having studied the other ingredients for successful reflection, reflection is not just thinking, mindlessly having fleeting thoughts about our day. It is a deliberate, considered process. The potential learning that can occur during the process of reflection is remarkable and can result in actions being taken, or future behaviours being altered, the influence of which will be felt by others, not just the reflector.

If we revisit the extended description of reflection, we can see where these two ingredients are situated. Indeed, unlike the previous ingredients, we can see that being process-orientated and deliberate underpin the whole of the extended description.

> *'Reflection is an essential, engaging process that allows the reflector to frame and reframe their reality that is, and has been experienced, moment by moment. Actively participating in the reflective process – that is, in, on or before an experience – requires us to tell our story and meander through that narrative, allowing ourselves to move where our thoughts and feelings wish to take us. It requires us to utilize skills of communication, to communicate with ourselves authentically, to become our own person-centred enquirer, understanding ourselves in relation to experiences we are about to have, are having or have had, empathically and with accuracy. Then stepping*

beyond the self and using this knowledge gained to understand how we may then have influenced those around us. To be fully immersed in this process, we must be open to learning about what constitutes 'I', leaving arrogance and complacency at the door, be kind and compassionate enough to offer ourselves unconditional positive regard, be actively engaged in mindfulness, and consciously aware of the self in our moments. Through a critical, analytical lens, we need to explore our experiences within the frame of how our history/background and current locus, culture and context influence who we are in our moments. Reflection requires us to open ourselves up to sourcing and learning new knowledge if the knowledge is not already known to us. And using that new knowledge gained to fill gaps in our current knowledge, challenge our preconceived notions and assumptions, and offer alternative ways of viewing experience to generate sense-making, thus creating information that can lead to personal and professional development. When we are fully open to and engaged in the process, reflection has the potential to empower us to be the best version of ourselves and inform our future experiences.'

Key points that can be taken from this chapter are:

- The notion of process underpins our reflection.
- Just as much learning can occur from the process of engaging in reflection as by understanding the outcome.
- The learning taken from the process is a pervasive form of learning that ensures a deep level of understanding.
- Reflection is a deliberate and considered process.
- Our actions and future behaviours because of reflection affect more than just ourselves.

Experience, Exploration, Sense-making, Implementation (EESI): a framework for reflection

---

Learning outcomes

By the end of this chapter, you will be able to:

- Decide upon the purpose and usefulness of reflective frameworks to support your reflections.
- Apply the reflective process as a new framework to support your engagement in reflection.
- Apply Brookfield's (2017) Four Lenses of Critical Reflection to the investigation and analysis of assumption in the reflective process.
- Appreciate how the EESI reflective framework is underpinned by the extended description of reflection and the ten essential ingredients.

The previous chapters have provided us with the knowledge we need to reflect, addressing how the ten essential ingredients connect to the extended description of reflection and support us to become effective reflective practitioners and the *best version of ourselves*. The chapters that follow this one will progress your use of reflection for different reasons by providing you with the knowledge required to reflect in the written format for academic purpose and through guided reflection in conversation. But before we move on, I want to support you in reflecting on and pre-experience – that is, after you have had your experience and prior to you having had that experience. I have purposefully left out reflecting in experience, or in-action as Schön (1983) called it, as personally I think this requires significant knowledge of reflection, significant reflective skills on your behalf, the critical awareness to be mindfully present and recognize inherent subjectivity and how it is influencing you in that very moment. But it is safe to say the more you practise reflecting on and before your experiences, the more proficient you will become at reflecting in experience.

In the first edition of this book, I included a chapter exploring some of the different reflective frameworks that have been published to support you to engage in the reflective process detailed in Figure 7.1 when reflecting for any purpose. It is not the intention of this chapter, however, to cover old territory but to move on from static frameworks that, in my humble opinion, can reduce the bespoke nature of reflection and create rigidity in the reflective process. As a result, this chapter will turn the process of reflection itself into a framework for reflection.

Have a go at the following exercise.

Exercise 7.1: Reflecting on your experience of using reflective frameworks

Reflect on your experience of using reflective frameworks/cycles/ models. Ask yourself:

- When have I used a reflective framework?
- Did I have a choice in the framework I used?
- What were my thoughts when using it?
- How did using it make me feel?
- Did I perceive it to be useful?
- Did it help me to engage in the reflective process as detailed in Figure 7.1?
- Would I use the same one(s) again?

In Chapter 1, I detailed in visual form what the reflective process is (see Figure 7.1).

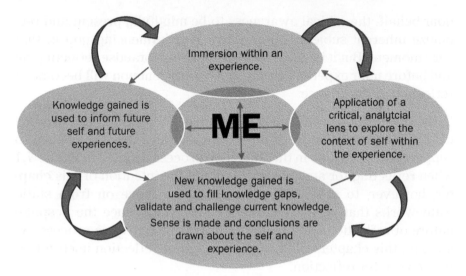

Figure 7.1 The reflective process

I have tried to highlight throughout this book that reflecting – whether on, in or before experience – is not formulaic. Yes, it is process-orientated and yes, it is deliberate, it is after all very purposeful, but it can also be messy. As we can see from Figure 7.1, all of the elements of the actual reflective process are interconnected with you/me/I at the absolute centre. The different aspects of this process can be moved between fluidly. In Chapter 9, I refer to it as 'meandering', and importantly only in the direction in which you wish to go. Sometimes you may move from describing your experience to sense-making, back to more description to help draw conclusions, then back to sense-making again and so on. Most importantly for reflection to occur and as a result successful reflective practice (which is using the knowledge gained to inform your future experiences), all aspects of the process need to be moved through for each and every experience you reflect on. So, when reflecting and engaging with the reflective process, give yourself permission to move with *your flow*. It is this process that I shall now turn into a reflective framework.

Experience, Exploration, Sense-making, Implementation – EESI

I think of the aspects of the reflective process detailed in Figure 7.1 as follows: immersion in and detailing the experience, a critical and analytical exploration of the experience, drawing conclusions to support sense-making, and implementation of that new knowledge to inform new experiences, with the resulting reflective framework thus being:

Experience, Exploration, Sense-making, Implementation – **EESI**

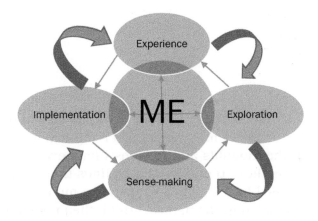

Figure 7.2 The EESI framework

However, we know from understanding the process of reflection identified in Figure 7.1, having knowledge of the ten essential ingredients, that the complexity of reflection is never quite demonstrated in any framework or acronym that represents that framework. Therefore, we will need support within the framework to ensure we are embodying the extended description of reflection and using those ten essential ingredients. We will need support to frame and reframe perception, to be open to learning, to communicate with ourselves to allow our authentic voice to be heard, and to explore how we are affected by culture, context, others and how we affect those around us to draw conclusions about who we are within our experiences to inform future self.

Have a go at the following exercise.

Exercise 7.2: Questions to support movement through and richness within each aspect of EESI

When reflecting on or pre-experience, what reflective questions and prompts do you think would be helpful to ask of yourself to support you to generate a richness of information for each of the aspects of EESI?

Experience ...
Exploration ...
Sense-making ...
Implementation ...

When I consider the *experience* aspect, I would want a framework to prompt and support me to remember my experiences, to be able to recall the thoughts and feelings I had, even recall what I may perceive as those thoughts and feelings that were insignificant. I would need to remember who was in my experience with me, how I responded to them, how I think they responded to me. I would want to remember the factors that influenced me and how I acted/behaved at that time. If I was reflecting prior to my experience, I would want questions within the framework to prompt me to consider and explore how I think and feel about the experience that I am about to have, how I may think and feel when the experience is occurring and why I think this way, what current knowledge I have about the experience, what I consider to be the factors that will influence my experience, who will be the significant others in my experience, and how I feel and think about that. I would want to be prompted to explore the potentiality of a future experience.

So now that we have our new reflective framework – **EESI** – I invite you to use the reflective prompts and questions in Tables 7.1 and 7.2 to help you develop your autonomy and knowledge of how to get the best out of each of the fours aspects for yourself. These are by no means exhaustive lists and I am sure you will have thought of some of your own when completing Exercise 7.2.

Table 7.1 Example reflective questions and prompts – *on experience*

Aspect	On experience
Experience	• What do you think happened? • Who/what else was in your experience with you? • How did you feel before/during/after? • What thoughts did you have before/during/after? • Did you have to prepare or behave in a certain way prior to the experience occurring? • Can you recall the atmosphere? Describe everything about it, even down to aromas you could smell. • Did anything stand out to you? • Where there any influencing factors? • How did you behave? • What did others do? • What do you think of others' behaviour?
Exploration	• What do I now think and feel about the experience? Why do I think and feel this way? • Was I influenced by my own value set, culture and context? Did I act in a manner consistent with my value set, culture and context? • How did my thoughts and feelings influence my behaviour? • What generated these thoughts and feelings within me? • Had I had previous experiences that influenced this particular experience? If so, in what way? • How do I think I affected those others in my experience, and why do I think this? • What are my thoughts on how I responded to others? Why do I think I responded the way I did? • How did other factors such as policy, politics, culture and context influence me in my experience? • What knowledge do I think I had about the experience? Did I utilize this knowledge appropriately? • Did I have enough knowledge? • Are there any different ways to view my experience? • What theory/literature is there that can help me to explore the experience? • How might another person in my experience describe their experience of me and my experience?
Sense-making	• What do I know about me now, my value set, my beliefs? • What conclusions can I draw about why I behaved the way I did? • What information do I have about how others received me/perceived me? • What information or themes have emerged because of this experience?

(continued)

Table 7.1 (Continued)

Aspect	On experience
Sense-making	• Is there anything I know now that I did not know before? • Is there anything I can do now that I could not do before? • What knowledge have I gained from reading the literature and theory? What does this tell me about the themes of my experience, and has it offered any new ways of viewing my experience? • Would I want to have experienced things differently? If so, in what way and why? • What conclusions can I draw about myself? • What conclusions can I draw from how other people would describe their experience of my experience?
Implementation	• How will what I now know inform my future experiences both professionally and personally? • Are there aspects of me that I would like to develop/embrace/change? If so, how will I do this? • Am I content with myself after this experience? If so, how can I maintain and translate this contentment to other areas of my life? • Am I content with how others view me? How will I maintain this or develop this? • What knowledge of any themes emerging would I wish to know more about? How will I gain this extra knowledge?

Table 7.2 Example reflective questions and prompts – *pre-experience*

Aspect	Pre-experience
Experience	• What do you think will happen? • Who/what else will be in your experience with you? • How do you feel about this? • What thoughts are you having about this experience? • Do you have to prepare to behave in a certain way? • What do you think the atmosphere will be like? Describe everything about it, even the things that might seem insignificant. • Does anything stand out to you? • Are there any influencing factors? • How do you think you will behave? • What do you think others will do? • What do you think of others' potential behaviours?
Exploration	• Why do I think and feel this way? • What is influencing my own value set, culture and context? Do I think I will act in a manner consistent with my value set, culture and context?

(continued)

Table 7.2 (Continued)

Aspect	Pre-experience
Exploration	• How do I think my thoughts and feelings will influence my behaviours? • What is generating these thoughts and feelings within me? • Are previous experiences influencing this experience? If so, in what way? • How do I think I will affect those others in my experience, and why do I think this? • What are my thoughts on how I might respond to others? Why do I think I might respond that way? • How will other factors such as policy, politics, culture and context influence me in my experience? • What knowledge do I think I have about the experience? How can I evidence this knowledge and utilize this knowledge appropriately? • Do I have enough knowledge? • Are there any different ways to view my experience? • What theory/literature is there that can help me to explore this experience? • How might another person in my experience describe the potentiality of the experience?
Sense-making	• What do I know about me now, my value set, my beliefs? • What conclusions can I draw about why I might behave the way I think I will? • What information do I have about how others may receive me/perceive me? • What information or themes have emerged because of this experience? • What do I know now that I did not know before? • Is there anything I can now do that I could not do before? • What knowledge have I gained from reading the literature and theory? What does this tell me about the themes of my experience? Has it offered any new ways of viewing my experience? • How would I now like to experience my experience? • What conclusions can I draw about myself? • What conclusions can I draw from how other people would describe their experience of my experience?
Implementation	• How will what I now know inform this future experience? • Are there aspects of me that I would like to develop/embrace/change? If so, how will I do this?

(continued)

Table 7.2 (Continued)

Aspect	Pre-experience
Implementation	• Am I content with what I have found out about me prior to this experience? • Am I content with how others may view me? How will I maintain this or develop this? • What knowledge of any emerging themes would I wish to know more about? How will I gain this extra knowledge? • How will I use this knowledge to inform this future experience?

How did what you wrote down as reflective prompts in Exercise 7.2 compare to the lists in Tables 7.1 and 7.2?

Have a go now at the following exercise where you are invited to write down an experience and immerse yourself in the first part of the reflective process using the reflective prompts under the **E** for experience.

Exercise 7.3: Describing your experience

Either write down or record a description of an experience you would like to recall or explore the potentiality of using the reflective prompts from the EESI under the **E** for experience.

● How did you find the prompts?
● Did they help you to describe the actual or prospective experience?
● Did they help you to immerse yourself in the experience?
● Was your voice authentic?
● Would you add any reflective prompts of your own?

Moving onto the next aspect of EESI, the second **E** as we know relates to the analytical exploration of the experience. The following is an extract from one of my student's reflective writing essays where Matron Tom is exploring his experience of a critical incident. Read the extract and circle where you can determine potential use of some of the prompts under the **E** for exploration.

Braillon and Taiebi (2020) suggest that active listening skills are easily overlooked but are cornerstones of communication and foster empathy. I embedded these skills, alongside communication facilitation techniques such as reflective of feeling, paraphrasing, use of open-ended questions, and therapeutic silence (Walsh-Burke, 2006). I know that my responses were well received as the family commented that they had felt listened to and had been shown empathy by allowing them to lead questioning and being attentive to their immediate needs as a griever. Staff reflected that empathy was evident in the way I had used open-ended questions, allowed time for response, and avoided sympathetic responses. On reflection, I can determine that some of my reactions were more sympathetic in nature; whilst it could be argued that this may resonate less meaningfully for others, it does show humanity, a trait that I have always tried to portray during my integrations with patients, as a way of them seeing that I am not doing care 'to them' rather that I am with them on the journey. There were times that I displayed a tangible emotional response. I now view this empathic response as part of my personality and attached less negative connotation to it. Thompson and Thompson (2008) believe it's recognized by many as 'human' as pure empathy is seldom possible, with some situations evoking an emotional response in us. Morse et al (1992) differentiate sympathy with empathy, whereby sympathy is an emotional response to the experience of another by absorbing the others' suffering to some extent. In contrast empathy is an objective view – a dispassionate glance yet motivated by deep concern for the other. I now recognize that when colleagues were showing emotional response to the experience, showing empathy involved me being emotionally aware, aware of what they are going through, without allowing the emotions to affect me, all of which enhanced my ability to sustain my leadership role and be more effective in debrief.

Could you determine if Matron Tom had used questions that required him to explore his values, his influence on others and how they responded to him? Does Matron Tom allow himself to have an authentic voice? I think we can read even in this brief extract that he is attempting to explore the experience so he can migrate into sense-making.

Now let's repeat this exercise for the next aspect of EESI, sense-making. Take a look at the second extract from Matron Tom and repeat the exercise. Circle where you perceive you can determine use of some of the reflective prompts under **S** for sense-making.

Looking back, I had multiple assumptions about how I expected staff may be feeling, the experience exposed emotional bias I held, and furthermore my need to display emotional intelligence whilst supporting colleagues within a reflective/debrief scenario. Thompson and Thompson (2008) propose that being tuned into other people's feelings, as well as those of my own and being able to read other's emotions, allows us to notice subtle cues in their language and behaviour, giving us important messages about their emotional state. I now recognize that there were times that I did not effectively acknowledge the emotional reactions of myself, or others, for example I held the assumption that (like me) this was their first experience of managing a death, and therefore they may be feeling similar emotions to me. Self-awareness is an important aspect of emotional intelligence. Goleman (2004: 88) describes it as 'the ability to recognise and understand your moods, emotions, and drives, as well as their effect on others', building on this saying we need to self regulate by controlling and redirecting disruptive impulses and moods. We should regulate our thinking process, suspend judgement before acting (Goleman, 2004) and aligned to self-regulation is that reflective practice is concerned with thinking about emotions and to act accordingly (Farrell, 2008). I was also suppositional in my view that everyone involved would want to revisit the event, naively positioning myself by prompting the conversation towards what happened. For some, this approach was cathartic and enabled a healthy outpouring of emotions, whilst for others it appeared less therapeutic and further traumatizing. Reflecting on my own emotions linked to this, I now think that there may have been some vicarious trauma playing out as we recounted the events in detail ... I now feel more confident in exploring my own emotions and less fearful of ridicule, or how I may be perceived as a leader. Fundamentally, this process has taught me how to pick up on emotional cues, reading body language and appropriate responses to trauma, whilst I recognize that I was in danger of having compassion fatigue because of helping others with their grief.

I think we can clearly see here that Matron Tom is in the sense-making phase. He is drawing conclusions about the experience, and he is gaining new knowledge about himself. He is also managing to challenge knowledge he thought was absolute.

The final aspect of EESI is the **I** for implementation. Let us take a final look at Matron Tom and another brief extract of his writing. As with the previous extracts, where do you perceive use of some of the reflective prompts under the **I** for Implementation.

> I now make time to access regular peer supervision with a fellow matron, this provides opportunities to review our approach to helping those that we supervise, whilst planning new inventive ways to engage staff in clinical focused supervision. Clinical supervision is often under performed in my experience and not given the respect that it warrants. May (2003: 61) sees it as 'an essential tool in the continued professional development of all nurses, whether newly qualified or senior level' with Butterworth et al (1996) backing May's view, adding that it not only supports nurses, but enhances patient care. This is something that I now make sure I find time for ... We now have 6 weekly reflective practice forums; these are clinically focused and accessible to all, ensuring there is a platform for staff to feel empathically supported whilst cultivating ideas and enable change for the service. My personal development continues through access to the aforementioned, the knowledge gained has assisted me in being adaptive to the needs of others, whilst ensuring I make time to recognize my own emotional needs. The experience has given me a reminder that to value others, you need to first value yourself. My in-depth learning about emotional intelligence has bolstered my understanding of how I manage my interpersonal relationships, remain compassionate, and support my colleagues.

I would suggest we can view here how Matron Tom is putting some of what he has learned into reflective practice, which has empowered him to make alterations and add new initiatives into his practice.

These brief extracts have helped us to see EESI in a written form of action. But don't forget, this framework can be used when reflecting for any purpose. Matron Tom was not only reflecting for self here, but also for an academic piece of work. This framework can be used just for self.

Consequently, we now have the new reflective framework of **E**xperience, **E**xploration, **S**ense-making, **I**mplementation (**EESI**), faithfully grown from the reflective process with helpful reflective prompts and questions to support our movement through it. However, as there are other reflective frameworks/models/cycles in the published literature, I will repeat the advice that I offered in the first edition of this book. Use a framework that you understand and are comfortable with if you feel you need to use one, and do not be afraid to use more than one.

I would like us to move on now to explore a way in which we can get into a greater level of exploration in the reflective process and ways in which we can attempt to explore our experiences from different angles and the perspectives of others in our experiences. We know the prompts in the EESI framework ask questions of us that require a depth of thinking, so what I discuss next will help you to get into some of that depth of thinking and exploration.

Brookfield's Four Lenses of Critical Reflection

Stephen Brookfield is a prominent educationalist and is a seminal writer on adult learning, critical theory, thinking and reflection in education. When relating reflection to teaching, he described reflection as:

> the sustained and intentional process of identifying and checking the accuracy and validity of our teaching assumptions. We all work from a set of orienting, stock assumptions that we trust to guide us through new situations. Some of these are explicit and at the forefront of our consciousness ... Other assumptions are much more implicit. Implicit assumptions soak into consciousness from the professional and cultural air around you. Consequently, they're often harder to identify.
> (Brookfield, 2017: 2)

It is clear that Brookfield wants us to recognize that in teaching, teachers are not always aware of those thoughts and feelings that drive their teaching, or of how the context of the teaching environment influences thoughts towards teaching practices. He wants us to know that reflection can unearth those covert processes that are influencing our way of *being* in practice. It is no different for the nursing and the health professions – when we reflect, we are striving to uncover those areas that influence us but of which we are unaware. We now know that when reflecting for any profession or experience, that we are trying to identify our notion of self and understand how this notion of self influences our experiences. We are striving to bring to the conscious and make sense of how the notion of self is influenced by culture, policy and context. It should also be clear from previous chapters that we need to step beyond ourselves to understand how we may have influenced those around us and how we in turn are influenced by them.

Brookfield (2017) advises us that the best way to identify and connect with these hidden and known assumptions is to view ourselves through four very specific lenses: the student's eyes, colleagues' perceptions, personal experience, and theory and research. The student here, of course, simply represents anyone in your area of professional practice or who you might be supporting, engaging with or caring for. So, for example, a student nurse may alter the student lens for a patient lens, or they could maintain the student lens if they are a staff nurse mentoring a nursing student; a teacher/lecturer will maintain the student lens, but the student lens could also become the client lens. This is an adaptable framework.

Let's consider the student lens. This lens asks us to obtain feedback from our students, our patients, etc. by attempting to see ourselves through their eyes. A common assumption Brookfield notes 'is that the meanings we ascribe to our actions are not always the same ones students take from them' (2017: 7). In our case, the meanings we attach to our communications and actions with our patients/clients may not be interpreted by them in the manner we intended. Obtaining feedback, or examining the responses of our patients to us, can help us to view ourselves through their eyes, and thus we can gain knowledge of how they interpret our caring. When I teach, I transparently encourage feedback. I am humble enough to know that not all my students respond to my teaching in the manner I assume they are. I invite verbal feedback and written anonymous feedback to encourage openness about their experiences of my teaching. Gaining their perspective can only enhance my understanding of self, which can only aid my teaching, which as a result can enhance my students' experience of learning. As a nurse, I paid attention to how my patients responded to me, to observe if their responses were expected based upon my behaviours towards them, and I would try and create ways of inviting feedback on their care so they did not feel as if they were 'put on the spot'. All this enhanced my understanding of self, which in turn enhanced my caring and practice.

Colleagues' perceptions are a way of gaining feedback on their observations of our experiences. They can offer their unique perspective on what they observed, helping us to see things we cannot see. In your case, your colleague could be a peer or a clinical supervisor/educator. These colleagues can help you to explore your experience from different angles. This takes us back to our opening chapter and Pooh Bear. Feedback from his best friend gave him a different perspective and new knowledge on his experience, which helped to reframe his thinking about his experience – that is, it gave him a different perspective. This also reminds us of the extended description of reflection we have been discussing in previous chapters, where we need to step beyond ourselves to determine how others experienced our experience. The personal experience lens is everything we have discussed in this book, and our narrative is something we will be exploring the importance of in the remaining chapters.

According to Brookfield, our final lens of theory and research 'can provide unexpected and illuminating interpretations of familiar as well as newly complex situations' (2017: 8). Let us recap my experience of using theory to illuminate a different interpretation of an experience I was having with a colleague. In Chapter 2, I described my experience of a boss who I would describe as a bully. I was struggling to make sense of why I was responding the way I was to this person. During a session with my mentor, I was advised to read some of the theory on transactional analysis before my next session with him. I was not sure as to why, but I did as suggested. The *light bulb* moment I experienced was life-changing. The theory that I read and digested helped to bring some objectivity into the subjective, it gave me a different perspective of my experience, and I was able to understand that I was responding as a frightened child to this 'bully' who was an angry adult. I was able to take this new information back to my facilitated reflection sessions. I was able to explore why I was a frightened child, unearthing information because of the theory that I read. As a result, I was able to inform my future experiences and alter my responses to my boss, and over time the ripple effect meant they altered their responses to me for the better. I was able to take control of my experiences.

Now go back and review Matron Tom's thoughts and see how he uses theory to support the exploration of his experience. The theory/literature provides knowledge that Matron Tom uses to achieve a deep level of exploration.

Have a go at the following exercise:

Exercise 7.4: Experiences of receiving feedback

In the final exercise of this chapter, jot down examples of where you have received feedback in any form, from your peers, tutors, patients, colleagues, etc. How did you experience the feedback? What thoughts and feelings did it leave you with? Did it help you to gain more information about you? Did it challenge any preconceived assumptions you may hold about yourself?

This chapter has provided us with a new framework for reflection – EESI – grown authentically from the reflective process itself. This will hopefully support the fluidity and meandering quality required in the reflective process. There are useful reflective prompts contained within the framework that will help your exploration. Viewing our experiences through the four different lenses also adds dimensions to the knowledge we can gain of self that we might not have gained through using just one lens of our personal experience.

The knowledge you have gained will support you in the final chapters of this book where we explore using another framework for reflection that has been specifically created to support your reflective writing in an academic setting, and where we will also explore how all the knowledge we have gained translates into guided reflection through conversation.

Key points that can be taken from this chapter are:

- There is more than one reflective framework, and the one you choose, if you decide to use one, ought to be the one you are most comfortable with.
- The reflective process can be utilized as a framework.
- EESI is a fluid framework that can be meandered through.
- Reflective prompts and questions will support engagement with EESI.
- The idea of Brookfield's Four Lenses of Critical Reflection will help you to view your experiences from different angles bringing some objectivity into the subjective.

Reflective writing – for self and academic purposes

Learning outcomes

By the end of this chapter, you will be able to:

- Give yourself permission to freewrite.
- Become comfortable using 'I' in your writing.
- Appreciate the broad concept of reflective writing.
- Use journaling as a mode of documenting the fluidity of the movie of your life.
- Judge the value of journaling as a method of showing movement through your experiences.
- Write reflectively for yourself and academia.
- Recognize the value the wonderful world of information in its broadest sense has in supporting sense-making of experience.
- Apply the reflective framework Experience, Deconstruction, Implementation (EDI) (Clarke, 2021) in supporting your reflective writing for academic assessment.

> Reflective writing can find out not only how and what we need to say, but also significantly *why*. Reflective writing captures events, individuals, thoughts, feelings and values; it can structure and illuminate them. Reflective practitioners write for self-illumination and exploration, not to create a product.
>
> (Bolton and Delderfield, 2018: 135–36)

In the previous chapters, we discussed in detail what reflection is and explored in some depth the essential ingredients required to reflect. I think we should now have a good grasp of the wonderful world of reflection and what skills and attitudinal qualities are required to be effective reflective practitioners. In Chapter 7, we were introduced to a new reflective framework that can support us to move through the reflective process fluidly and authentically. It is the intention of this chapter to examine reflection through the mode of reflective writing for self, for academic and professional purposes. The chapter will explore the differences between the three, it will introduce journaling as a way of freewriting to document the progression of experience that may otherwise not be captured, and it will guide you through using another, yet very specific framework created to purposefully support reflective writing for academic purposes.

Reflective writing for differing purposes

Have a go at completing the following exercise.

Exercise 8.1: Experiences of reflective writing

What immediate thoughts and feelings do you have about reflective writing? Now think about when you have written reflectively before. Use the following prompts to help you immerse yourself in that previous experience:

- When you reflected in the written format, what were your thoughts about it at the time?
- When you wrote reflectively, was it for a particular purpose?
- Were you allowed to use 'I'?
- How did you find writing reflectively, and why was it like this for you? Enjoyable? Hard/easy? Stressful? Cathartic? Lacking clarity?
- Knowing what you now know, when asked to write reflectively, would you describe what you were being asked to do as reflective or evaluative writing?

Reflective writing for any purpose, whether for personal, professional or academic reasons, requires the use of, and will be underpinned by, all ten essential ingredients for successful reflection, and most importantly an accurate understanding of reflection as provided in Chapter 1. It will also require you to move through the reflective process we have detailed in prior chapters. Reflective writing, just as when reflecting in a conversation guided by another (something we shall discuss in the following chapter), in a group situation or on our own in purposeful, quiet, thoughtful contemplation, requires a genuine curiosity about self, a willingness to investigate and an openness to challenge perspective, assumptions, beliefs and ideas.

There are, however, some differences in writing reflectively for self, professional and academic purposes.

Exercise 8.2: Writing reflectively for self, professional and academic purposes

What might the differences be between these three forms of writing reflectively? Are there any similarities between them?

When writing reflectively for academia and professional practice, you may have been and will be asked to evaluate what you did well and not so well. This is a reductionist view of reflection and in health, education and life sciences, a misunderstood view. But if this is a requirement of an assessment brief – even if we know it is not really requiring us to reflect appropriately – it is advisable to follow the brief you are given.

When writing reflectively for academic purposes, you may also be required to be *critically reflective*, or to *critically reflect on*, or *to provide a piece of critical reflection*. By asking this, your lecturers/module leaders are trying to 'describe a quality in writing where the reader [you] can see that the writing comes from careful thinking … and you are moving up the stairway of critical thinking' (Williams et al., 2012: 12). It is important to remember that whatever your lecturer wishes to term reflective writing, reflection in any form should be deliberate, rigorous, exploratory and analytical. I would argue – and maybe you would too having read the previous chapters – that we cannot fully engage in the reflective process without being critically analytical.

Nonetheless, when writing reflectively for professional purposes or self, you are not being assessed against rigid academic criteria. When writing for academia, you will be expected to draw upon theory and to utilize the literature within your writing, and you may well be marked according to whether you have indeed read widely and used theory appropriately. However, information gleaned from the academic literature, guidelines/policy documents and so on is invaluable when reflecting for *any* purpose. Engaging with factors outside of yourself such as this can bring some objectivity into the subjective, can enable you to view your experiences from different perspectives, can challenge your thinking and your view of the world, and fill gaps in your knowledge, even when not being assessed against academic criteria.

Take a look at Table 8.1, which lists the requirements for reflective writing for different purposes. As you can see across the three forms of reflective writing, there are subtle differences, and these differences are really influenced by the context in which you are asking yourself or being asked to reflect.

Table 8.1 The three forms of writing reflectively

Academic	*Professional*	*Personal*
Intent of writing		
• Validates your narrative/story	• Validates your narrative/story	• Validates your narrative/story
• Generates knowledge about what constitutes 'I'	• Generates knowledge about what constitutes 'I'	• Enables you to hear your own voice authentically
• Generates self-awareness	• Generates self-awareness	• Enables you to observe personal growth
• Supports the growth of emotional intelligence	• Supports the growth of emotional intelligence	• Generates knowledge about what constitutes 'I'
• Enables understanding of use of self within therapeutic relationships	• Enables understanding of use of self within therapeutic relationships	• Generates self-awareness
		• Supports the growth of emotional intelligence
• Enables understanding of how you respond to people and how people respond to you	• Enables understanding of how you respond to people and how people respond to you	• Enables understanding of use of self in any relationship
		• Enables understanding of how you respond to people and how people respond to you
• Closes the theory-practice gap	• Closes the theory-practice gap	• Enhances understanding of a subject related to personal matters
		• Empowers you to inform future experiences

(continued)

Table 8.1 (Continued)

Academic	Professional	Personal
• Enhances understanding of a subject • Supports application of theory to practice • Empowers you to inform future experiences • Meet the requirements of an assessment brief • Helps pass a module • Creates a product	• Enhances understanding of a subject related to practice • Supports application of theory to practice • Empowers you to inform future experiences • Meets the requirements of professional body standards and revalidation processes • Creates a product	

Writing style

Academic	Professional	Personal
• Uses 'I' • Organized • Professional language • Academic language • Personal language used in a thoughtful manner • Well structured • Formatted in accordance with a prescription • Free hand • Computer • Dictated • Spelling, punctuation, grammar is highly important	• Uses 'I' • Organized • Professional language • Personal language used in a thoughtful manner • Well structured • Formatted dependent upon context • Free hand • Computer • Dictated • Spelling, punctuation, grammar is highly important	• Uses 'I' • Messy • Personal language used • Unstructured • Lacks formatting • Free hand • Computer • Dictated • Spelling, punctuation, grammar not of concern

Uses literature/theory/evidence

Academic	Professional	Personal
• Explicitly • Wide range of reading on the themes for the module demonstrated	• Explicitly • Wide range of reading on the themes in practice	• Explicitly • Wide range of reading on the themes of what has been chosen to reflect on • Used to bring objectivity into the subjective

(continued)

Table 8.1 (Continued)

Academic	*Professional*	*Personal*
• Used to bring objectivity into the subjective • Used to confirm and challenge thinking about the themes/subject being reflected upon • Used to provide different perspectives • Used to demonstrate and explore the thinking of others in the world of information • Used to fill gaps in knowledge • Used to support the synthesis of ideas and drawing of conclusions related to the assessment brief • Correct referencing style used dependent upon the requirements of the higher education setting	• Used to bring objectivity into the subjective • Used to confirm and challenge thinking about the practice themes/subject being reflected upon • Used to provide different perspectives • Used to demonstrate and explore the thinking of others in the world of information • Used to update knowledge • Used to fill gaps in knowledge • Used to support the synthesis of ideas and drawing of conclusions about self and practice • Correct referencing style used dependent upon what the reflector knows	• Used to validate/confirm and challenge thinking about the themes/subject being reflected upon • Used to provide different perspectives • Used to demonstrate and explore the thinking of others in the world of information • Can be therapeutic/affirming • Used to fill gaps in knowledge • Used to draw conclusions about personal thoughts and feelings • Referencing might be used, or notes made of where information has been gathered from as a record to refer to for future reference

The power of narrative

Before we take a closer look at reflective writing for academic purposes, I would like us to explore the power of narrative and the first aspect of the reflective process – immersion in the experience. I suggested in Chapter 1 that this is possibly the most important aspect of the reflective process. This is the aspect of the reflective process that powerfully validates our thoughts and feelings, by empowering us to take the time out to explore the movie of our life and to empathically acknowledge this movie (Clarke, 2021). This is also the aspect that when writing for academic purposes, which is ultimately about product creation against rigid criteria, will not have much importance given over to it. Yet as I have already stated, this is the most important aspect of the reflective process because without it, beyond the reasons already mentioned, critical exploration cannot occur.

> We do not 'store' experience as data, like a computer: we story it.
> (Winter, 1988: 235)

Immersing ourselves in our experiences and writing about it requires use of the factual and personal storylines. The factual storyline is the plot, the physical story, the description of what you did, how you behaved during your day, how you woke up, what you did next (e.g. brushed your hair, cleaned your teeth, walked the dog). Those of you who remember the Indiana Jones movies and the early James Bond films, these are examples of movies told almost exclusively from the frame of the factual storyline (Tobin, 2019) – vivid description of action where the personal frame is not needed. In contrast, according to Tobin (2019), the film 'Rocky' manages to successfully incorporate an account of Rocky's experience from both the factual and personal storylines. Factual in the sense of will he train hard enough, learn enough technique, learn to punch harder; personal in the sense of will he overcome his insecurities, will he find love, happiness – we see the growth of Rocky as a person in the film (Tobin, 2019). In the telling of the story of experience, which is the set of scenes, the plot, the sub-plots, the characters within the story, the start/middle/end (Bolton and Delderfield, 2018), the narrative becomes the driving force of how the story is told, and the perspective from which the story will unfold.

The narrative in reflective writing is autobiographical in nature. So, when we write the story of our experience, the narrative of that story will be written from the perspective of 'I'. Because it is our story, we choose the plot, we choose the sequence of events to discuss, we choose the perspective from which we tell the story because we are the central character. But this also allows us to narrate our story from different perspectives. We can tell the story from the stance of any one of the different roles we play in life, and we can narrate the story from the perspectives of the different characters in it.

Therefore, narrative has the power through the telling and retelling of our stories through these different lenses, to generate different information and give us new ways of understanding our experiences.

Freewriting and journaling

To narrate the story of our lived experience, we need to learn to give ourselves permission to write freely, without thinking, without order. To allow the story to come to you and through you without constriction (Bolton, 2010). Put simply, this means giving yourself permission to think, feel, recollect and transfer those thoughts, feelings and recollections to paper.

Students and staff I speak to find reflective writing incredibly difficult. Students, for example, are often told by academic staff not to use 'I', 'as it is considered less academic to do so'. And many staff who are required to engage in continuing professional development and to write reflectively were told the same during their own undergraduate days, and as a result tell their own students not to use 'I'. Yet, if you were to undertake a doctorate (level 8) and engage in qualitative research, you would be expected in your thesis to use 'I' to demonstrate reflexivity within your research. So, use of 'I' does not reduce the academic quality of the writing. But we do at times need to give ourselves permission to use it.

So, before we move on to writing for academic purposes, have a go at the following two exercises. The first, the six-minute write, is adapted from Bolton (2010), who sees writing as 'a gift to yourself' and I would agree. This is an adaptation of stage 1 of Bolton's *Through the Mirror Writing* and is the first stage in giving yourself permission to connect mind to hand to paper and use 'I'.

Exercise 8.3: The six-minute write – but use 'I' from start to finish

Write whatever is in your head, uncensored. What are you thinking right now? How do you feel right now?

Write without stopping for six minutes.

Don't stop to think or be critical, even if it seems rubbish.

Allow it to flow with **no thought for spelling, grammar** or **proper form**.

Give yourself permission to **write anything**. You need not even reread it.

Whatever you write will be **right**: it is yours, and no-one else has to read it.

But give yourself permission to use 'I'.

Source: Adapted from Bolton (2010: 107–8).

How did you find just writing? I know when I first tried it, I found it hard. I felt silly and struggled to think of what to write about. But once I stopped overthinking it and just let my head connect to my hand, I found it quite liberating.

You may find the next exercise, which a colleague kindly introduced me to, slightly easier as I am going to give you a topic to write about. Again, give yourself permission to write freely.

Exercise 8.4: Your name!

Write down uncensored whatever you want to say about your name.

Write without stopping for as long as you wish to write for.

Use 'I'.

You can use the following as prompts – but just write, don't overthink:

● Do you like your name?
● What thoughts do you have about your name?
● What memories do you have of your name?
● What have people said about your name?
● What have been your nicknames over the years?
● What does your name say about you?

Here we are just trying to allow our emotions and thoughts to connect to the paper through the hand – if you don't like freewriting, then use a recording device and transcribe your thoughts into a Word document. In reflective writing, we need to give ourselves permission to be present with ourselves so that use of 'I' becomes natural and to let the narrative flow, so that it is not contrived.

One way to empower ourselves to connect with and use 'I' authentically is to 'journal'. Journaling is a means of recording that uses writing, notes, drawings, colour, pictures and so on to express how we are feeling and what we are experiencing on a daily, weekly, monthly or whatever basis you like. If you recount the film 'Bridget Jones's Diary', you will remember that it is the main character who makes journaling pretty fashionable. Journaling is a very personal and simple, yet powerful way of connecting organically, authentically and without constraint to the power that is our narrative and then expressing this. Journaling is not constrained by the requirements of academia or meeting professional body standards, it is truly freewriting, where you can validate *you* empathically. Journaling is also private, and something you can choose not to share with anyone else.

Take a look at Box 8.1 where the benefits of journaling are listed.

Box 8.1: The benefits of journaling

- Always available – never too busy
- It never answers back – it's always open to listening
- It maintains privacy and confidentiality
- It opens up a continuous relationship with the self
- It accepts everything and everyone unconditionally
- It does not get tired of hearing the same thing over and over again
- It can be written in the moment and therefore a true reflection of your thoughts and feelings
- It gives you a chance to communicate with yourself
- It brings greater clarity through the process of reflective writing
- It never disagrees with you
- It provides a record of learning and development

Source: Brockbank and McGill (2006: 283–84).

Johns (2010) also sees the benefits of journaling as he believes that this mode of freewriting gives us a voice to privately express ourselves, and because of the privacy that journaling can provide, it can also support our ability to be honest with self. He suggests it is a way to override the censorship that can occur when we are conscious of how others may perceive and receive us. Engaging with the first aspect of the reflective process and immersing ourselves in our experiences in this mode, writing freely and without thought and consideration for how others might perceive us is, as I said earlier, liberating.

Importantly, journaling can document progress, which I did not understand the true power of until I used it myself when I experienced an especially difficult event in my life. When I had my experience each evening before sleeping, I wrote in the tiniest of notebooks what I thought and felt about what had happened to me. I never showed anyone. I used my journal as a way of authentically expressing myself with absolutely no filter. I think the air at times may have turned blue with the words I used to express myself. I didn't move through the process of reflection – I remained in the first part. I immersed myself in recalling my experience and my thoughts and feelings about it. There was a moment a year later when I was feeling particularly bad, I thought I was not moving forward, I felt static in my thoughts and feelings, but that night instead of writing in my journal I decided to read it. Reading it was revealing for me. I noticed as I was reading how many months had passed since my first entry, and that I was not writing in it every night now. I noticed the air was no longer turned blue with the way I needed to express myself. I noticed that I had started to document happier thoughts and that I was feeling different, less angry, less upset. My journal had documented the movie of my life for me, my narrative over the 12 months showed me how far I had moved on in my healing journey. My journal demonstrated to me that I was able to think of other things now, that my experience was no longer all-consuming. This was a very powerful moment for me. I had not analysed anything about my experience, that would be for a later date, when I was ready, but journaling my experience, allowing myself to express what constituted 'I', freely and without judgement, showed me how much I had moved on when I thought I had not.

Although there are lots of downloadable journal templates that you can access, please don't think you need to follow a prescribed format. If you choose to journal, simply connect with yourself, as you did in the first exercise in this chapter. Use whatever you need to connect with yourself, for example you may decide to write in pink, red or yellow. You may decide to express yourself by cutting out pictures from magazines. You could choose to immerse yourself in a very particular experience, or you could just immerse yourself in how you feel and what you are thinking at that very specific moment in time – importantly, it is your journal, no-one need ever see it, so it doesn't matter. But look at Box 8.2, where there are some non-prescriptive prompts to help you get started.

Box 8.2: Prompts to support journaling

- What do I want to write about?
- What has happened today/this week?
- How do I feel right now?
- Is this different to how I have felt today?
- What thoughts am I having right now?
- Have I been thinking like this all day?
- Is this how I want to feel?
- Are these the thoughts that I want right now?
- What do I think about others around me?
- How do I think others have experienced me today?
- Is there anything I need to pay attention to from what I am writing here?
- Do I want to share this with anyone?

Now that you have given yourself permission to use 'I' and taught yourself to connect with you, take a look at Exercise 8.5.

Exercise 8.5: Have a go at journaling

Grab whatever you need to start. I know I needed a really funky looking notebook and some colourful pens. I also needed glitter in my pens! What you use is personal to you.

Now give yourself permission to be present with yourself and write about anything you want, for as long as you want to. But make sure to note how you are feeling and what you are thinking. Do this as often as you feel you want to. This is great practice for when you need to connect with *you* when reflecting and when you will need to immerse yourself in an experience and reflect on it for academic purposes.

Now that we can freewrite and are comfortable using 'I', let us move on to reflective writing for academic purposes.

Reflective writing for academic purposes, using Experience, Deconstruction, Implementation (EDI)

As you may be aware from the first edition of this book, all of the principles of academic writing also underpin reflective writing for academic purposes. Here, I do not wish to revisit those principles in the same manner but would instead like to show you how to use a very specific framework that supports reflective writing explicitly for academic purposes. To be honest, for several years I had been unhappy about students being pushed into using Gibbs' reflective cycle as a structure to write reflectively for an academic essay. I felt that using Gibbs in a vertical sense, overly fractured work and disconnected the academic story being told. As a result, it took me nearly a year to create a framework that would specifically support you to reflect for the purpose of nailing the requirements of an assessment brief on your course. And so EDI was created and published in the *Journal of Reflective Practice* in 2021.

EDI comprises three very distinct sections – **E**xperience, **D**econstruction, **I**mplementation – with prompts in each section that move you through the reflective process and also support you to ensure your reflective writing is academically sound and underpinned by all the principles that were discussed in the first edition. You should be able to see the similarities between EDI and EESI, the principles of which were introduced and discussed in the previous chapter. Whereas we can use EESI to reflect in any mode, EDI is specifically formulated to support reflective writing for academic purposes.

Let us now look at each section of EDI as you may find this helpful if you choose to use this framework when writing reflectively for academic purposes.

Experience

The *experience* section of EDI will help you to immerse yourself in the first part of the reflective process and in writing the movie of your experience, the important narrative that we have been discussing. Your assignment brief will no doubt prescribe an experience to reflect on, either by telling you what type of experience to recall or giving you a topic to reflect on. One thing you will need to consider when writing reflectively for academic purposes is that most marks are awarded for demonstrating adherence to the academic principles of structure, analysis, wider reading, use of theory, etc., so for academic reflective writing, this section will need to be one of the shortest parts of your essay. My advice to you, though, is do not overly concern yourself about the word count initially. When you do your detailed editing before you submit your work, this is where you can cut down your words by identifying repetition, waffle, content that is not required and so on. The experience section, however, is a difficult piece to write well, as you are trying to give your marker a view into your world, which is not necessarily an easy thing to do.

You should be able to determine from the prompts that this section gives you permission to use 'I', it does not require you to get into any analysis but instead describe your experience without feeling the need to use any theory. This is the part of your story that is factual and personal. Most importantly, own your thinking, feeling and behaviours.

Box 8.3: *Experience*, Deconstruction, Implementation

Experience: Paint the picture of your experience (observe yourself in your experience or watch your own film – then relay this narrative to your marker/reader).

- Where did the experience occur? Introduce the setting or context.
- What happened?
- What were your Thoughts, Feelings and Behaviours? Those of others?
- What happened next?
- How did this affect/alter your Thoughts, Feelings, Behaviours and those of others?

The marker/reader should feel as if they were there with you in your experience.

A descriptive factual section. There is no need for interpretation, assumptions, deconstruction, analysis or literature in this section. Own your feelings and thoughts on what you were part of.

Source: Adapted from Clarke (2021).

Take a look at the following two extracts of a student writing about their experience of a physiotherapy placement, then have a go at the exercise.

Exercise 8.6: Which of two extracts conveys the experience reflectively?

Extract 1

When working with the physiotherapist, watching closely it was safe to assume they understood the needs of the patient. Their assessment of the patient was thorough, and they took an excellent medical history. Using skills of being person-centred the team communicated and connected with the patient in order to understand their unique needs in order to formulate a plan to support the patient in their rehabilitation and recovery. The patient felt heard and understood. As the student it then became okay to become part of the assessment process.

Extract 2

I spent the morning working closely with the lead physiotherapist. I was anxious at first as I had not observed this person previously and I was usure of how to act and what I would be allowed to contribute. So my default was to just initially observe as I did not want to get in their way. I observed how they communicated with one particular patient. At the time I thought that their assessment of the patient was thorough, and I thought they took an excellent medical history. The senior physiotherapist to me did not appear to want to rush, this is because I saw how they took their time with the patient, I felt that they spoke clearly and seemed to give plenty of time for question and answers. Remembering what I was taught about being person-centred I felt that the patient may have felt heard and understood and at the centre of their care. Seeing how relaxed the patient was and how natural I thought the physiotherapist was with them, gave me confidence to ask the patient questions about their injury. I wanted to become part of the assessment rather than just an observer. Just observing does make me feel uncomfortable as if I am just a voyeur.

Now answer the following questions:

● Why is extract 2 following the structure and the prompts provided in the *experience* aspect of the framework?
● What would need to happen with extract 1 to make it more reflective?
● What are the deficiencies of extract 1 that prevent it from being reflective?

We can see in extract 1 that there is no use of 'I', the person reflecting does not place themselves in their experience at all. What the person reflecting observed is also not owned as a personal thought or feeling. The thoughts and feelings are written as statement of fact (e.g. 'they took an excellent medical history'). This is not written as though it were the personal thinking of the student; it has been written as a known fact. However, this is a personal thought and cannot be confirmed; until the student reflecting uses theory to gain knowledge on what they have observed, they cannot know if their thinking about what they observed is accurate. Extract 1 demonstrates a more evaluative impersonal style of writing, rather than reflective writing.

Deconstruction

The *deconstruction* section of EDI will help you to move from describing your narrative to a more analytical exploration of your experience, while helping you to stay connected to the purpose of the assessment brief – which as we know is one of the most important principles of academic writing. This section provides you with the acronym PEE (**P**oint, **E**vidence, **E**xploration) and prompts that begin with the letter **W** to support the construction of paragraphs that are analytical in their narrative. As you can see, the acronym asks you to create an opening to your paragraph that creates a *point* about your experience that connects it to the assessment brief; it then asks you to use the *evidence* of your experience and all the amazing literature to *explore* your experience using the extra prompts to usher you into a deeper level of exploration.

Box 8.4: Experience, *Deconstruction*, Implementation

Deconstruction of the experience that is positioned within the litera-ture. Provide an introductory paragraph that tells the marker/reader that the deconstruction (analysis) of the experience will occur against the purpose of the assignment brief.

Construct the rest of this section from paragraphs that use the **PEE** as detailed below and where appropriate use the prompts highlighted under the **E** for **E**xploration. These prompts are not prescriptive but when used can support the deconstruction of the experience and will help you to create paragraphs that are analytical in nature.

Create each paragraph in the main body of the essay from **PEE, W×7** and **c**.

- **P** = create a **P**oint about the experience that connects the expe-rience to the assignment brief.
- **E** = use the **E**vidence that is your experience (and other experi-ences if appropriate) and the literature to:

E = **E**xplore the meaning and the implications of your **P**oint by asking and then answering the following questions:

- **W**hy is this important? (Objective)
- **W**hy do I care about this? (Subjective)
- **W**hat are the connections between this point and the assignment brief? (Wider picture)
- **W**hat other perspectives/views are there of this? (Objective)
- **W**hat are the implications of this, for me/others/subject matter? (Subjective/Objective/Wider picture)
- **W**hat does this tell me about me, how I affect other people, how other people affect me? (Subjective)
- **W**hat does this tell me about the subject matter? (Objective / Wider picture)

c = **C**onclude the paragraph. What is the relevance of this discussion to the assignment brief, how does it connect? (Wider picture)

Finally, draw this section to a close by drawing a **C**onclusion that details what this has taught me about:

● Me
● Others
● How others perceive me
● The subject matter of the assignment brief; relate this back to the literature/evidence you have already laid down.

Source: Adapted from Clarke (2021).

Now have a go at the following exercise.

Exercise 8.7: Can you see the deconstruction?

Read the following extract where a student is exploring their experience of being with a patient who was worried about having a natural birth.

Empathy is one of the most important components in therapeutic work and supports having a person-centred approach that demonstrates understanding an individual's feelings and situation, through their own unique perspective (Rogers, 1980). Haley et al. (2017) advised that enhanced self-awareness and active listening can lead to improved empathy, which in turn improves patient-centred care. When I was asked to care for Jayne during my placement time, I perceived that I had been self-aware enough to leave my own thoughts and feelings to one side and I had truly attempted to get to know Jayne and had consistently tried to see the world through her eyes. I gave her an atmosphere of acceptance which Miller and Rollnick (2002) suggested is for inviting exploration, and I thought I had not assumed to give advice but instead encouraged her to openly discuss her fear of giving birth naturally. However, when I took time to consider Jayne's response to me, I became aware that I was not as accepting as I first thought and that my lack of self-awareness in the moments with Jayne had inhibited my empathic regard. According to Kirk (2007) empathy is understanding the perspective of another; however, by assuming to know how Jayne felt and comparing Jayne's experience with my own,

I had lost my ability to be empathic. My lack of self-awareness in this instance had inhibited my ability to connect with my own thoughts and feelings and as Dasilveira (2015) advises know them well enough to put to one side. Jayne on reflection had responded to me not necessarily negatively, we were able to chat and engage, but I think now she ceased being open with me as I had ceased being person-centred. I can recall now that she moved our conversation to the more trivial aspects of the day. On recollection my lack of empathy had pushed me into giving advice and this at that time was not what Jayne had needed. She needed me to actively listen and align with what Arnold (2014) suggested as being present enough to really hear and understand Jayne from her unique perspective. It can therefore be suggested that in order to be empathic and to be present enough to offer person-centred care, I will need to always be aware of myself in the moment and employ what Schön (1983) described as reflection in action. This will then allow me to be mindful of how my thoughts and feelings are affecting the experiences I have with patients and will allow me to respond accordingly.

Now, attempt the following:

- Highlight the parts of the extract that are showing use of the deconstruction phase of the framework.
- Circle or highlight the point being made.
- Circle or highlight the use of the theory.
- Circle or highlight the exploration of the experience using some of the prompts.

We can determine from this extract that the student reflecting has explored the meaning of self-awareness, its relationship to empathy and how all these elements combined support being person-centred. It also appears that they did learn a little about themselves, so we can see deconstruction of an aspect of their experience.

Good academic writing always requires paragraphs to have bookends, of openings and closings. The closings are what I call mini conclusions that close down the discussion in each paragraph. If you take a further look at the deconstruction phase, you will see that this also offers ideas on how to use those small conclusions in constructing the more traditional, larger conclusion that would, in a non-reflective essay, complete your piece of work. But as we now know, there is another aspect to the process of reflection, which is how we will use the conclusions we have drawn moving forwards.

Implementation

In a standard non-reflective piece of work, you would have finalized your writing with your conclusion to the deconstruction section. However, based on what we have discussed to this point, we know that there is one more aspect to the reflective process. We know the conclusions we draw from reflecting can teach us something new about ourselves or confirm what we already knew to be true. It is important in reflective writing for academic purposes to consider what you will do with what you have learned about yourself and the topic of the assessment brief. Your marker will want to know how you will use what you have learned to inform your future professional practice, and may even require a smart goal. So, ensure you treat the final section of your essay with as much care and importance as the first two aspects.

The prompts in the implementation section will enable you to consider and tell your marker what you will do with the wonderful knowledge you have gained from reflecting.

Box 8.5: Experience, Deconstruction, *Implementation*

Implementation: This final section will finalize your reflective piece and should be treated with as much consideration as the previous two sections. Although not as long as the deconstruction phase, it is no less significant.

Inform the reader/marker of:

● How this will inform your future self.
● How this will inform your future experiences.
● How this will inform your future practice/profession.

- What might you do to develop your personage and your professional you? (Again you can still position this final discussion in the literature, use the evidence to help support your assertions/opinions.)
- Finally, explain what the meaning/relationship of all of this is to the assignment brief.

Source: Clarke (2021).

Now have a go at the following exercise.

Exercise 8.8: Let's implement what we have learned

Think of an experience you have already reflected on. This can be any experience and any occasion that has required you to reflect. Follow the prompts in the implementation section and see if you can construct a paragraph that allows you to consider what you will do with what you have learned from reflecting.

Before I conclude this chapter, a final word on the use of literature when writing reflectively for academic purposes. You might already know from the previous edition of this book that the use of theory in academic and reflective writing can:

- create discussion;
- develop discussion;
- create debate;
- expand on points we have made;
- offer alternative viewpoints;
- enable things to be viewed from a different perspective;
- demonstrate we have engaged with the evidence and the literature that is out there;
- demonstrate that we can understand what we are reading;
- provide credibility to discussions we wish to develop;
- demonstrate we can understand the different types of evidence and how they should be used appropriately. (Clarke, 2017: 712)

But it can also bring some objectivity into the subjective. It is hoped that Exercise 8.7 helped you see how to use the literature appropriately in reflective writing. So, take a look at the following sentence:

> "'I believe I adopted a person-centred approach"
>
>   (Rogers, 1959).'

What is not right about how the reference has been used here? Here the person has used the reference as if Rogers were standing next to them and was able to confirm their personal thought that they adopted a person-centred approach. What educators would prefer to read is an 'exploration of what the students perceived they did that was person centred, aligned with, compared with, and contrasted against the theory of what Rogers and other authors would suggest is person centred' (Clarke, 2021). So, ensure you are not using the theory as an afterthought; instead, that you are using the theory to explore and generate meaning from your experience.

This chapter has explored reflective writing for personal, professional and academic purposes. We have acknowledged the need to use 'I' in reflective writing and we focused our efforts in recognizing the power of narrative and journaling. Furthermore, we have discovered how to use the EDI reflective framework to support construction of reflective writing for academic purposes.

Key points that can be taken from this chapter are:

- Reflective writing comes in different forms for different purposes.
- Freewriting is a useful way of enabling the use of 'I' and exploring our narrative, deeply and freely.
- Writing for self can be unstructured and uncensored.
- Journaling is a powerful tool to support the telling of our narrative and documenting progression.
- The principles that underpin academic writing also underpin reflective writing for academic purposes.
- Using a framework such as EDI can help us develop our ability to write reflectively for academic purposes.
- Literature has an important part to play in enabling and supporting the analysis of experience.

Guided reflective conversation

Learning outcomes

By the end of this chapter, you will be able to:

● Recognize what a reflective conversation should be and what it should not be.
● Know what a reflective conversation should look like for you, as the person receiving guided reflection.
● Know what to look for in a person who you allow to facilitate reflection in you.
● Discuss and apply what attitudinal qualities you will need to receive guided reflection.
● Describe the principles of Socratic questioning and apply these to the reflective conversation.
● Clarify what skills are required in order to offer guided reflection to someone.
● Apply the knowledge gained to practise facilitating and guiding reflection in another person.

In the previous chapter, we explored reflection through the mode of writing, a way of reflecting that will always be a solo activity unless we allow someone to view what we have written, for example a reflective essay in academic work for which we will receive feedback from our assessors, or the advice of a trusted friend. Chapter 5 showed us that reflecting alone has its limitations, and at no point within this book will I suggest that engaging in reflection is easy. We have learned about the significant skills and attitudinal qualities you will require to be able to fully engage in the reflective process. But even with all these skills, combined with bravery, open-mindedness, etc., and the tools discussed in Chapter 7 that can propel us into the criticality required for deep exploration, without another person supporting facilitation of reflection within us, it can remain difficult to put aside purposeful time to reflect and gain the level of criticality for that deep level of investigation into self.

The aim of this chapter, therefore, is to explore with you the experience of reflecting when being guided by another through reflective conversation. This chapter will help you to understand what it should feel like to be a part of a guided reflective conversation. It will help you to understand what qualities to look for in someone *you allow* to guide you through reflecting on your experiences and it will help you to also know what skills the facilitator of reflection possesses. By the end of this chapter, not only will you know what it should be like to be facilitated in reflecting on your experiences, but you will know enough about the skills and qualities to start to be able to support your peers, friends and eventually colleagues in their need to reflect on experience.

The guided reflective conversations you will have as part of your professional practice will usually be some form of professional/clinical supervision. As Driscoll noted, clinical supervision legitimizes and gives us permission to take time out to reflect on practice and to 'stop and think in the midst of practice (2000: 17). He further advised that 'not all reflective practice is clinical supervision, but all clinical supervision is reflective practice' (2000: 21). Therefore, I would suggest that during your training and during your professional career, you will at many points be on the receiving end of a guided reflective conversation. So, we can safely say it is important to know what this is and how it should be experienced.

Now, for those of you that have read the first edition of this book as well as this edition up to this point, you will have significant knowledge of reflection, what it is, its purpose, its importance and how to reflect alone. You will understand the skills and attitudinal qualities required to be an effective reflective practitioner. I would go as far as to say that you now have insider knowledge and potentially more knowledge than some who will try and develop reflection within you. So, knowing what you now know, have a go at the following exercise.

Exercise 9.1: What is a guided reflective conversation?

Jot down what you think a guided reflective conversation should be. What do you think it should *not* be? You can come back to this later and compare what you have written here to what you will learn in the following pages.

Take a look at the speech bubbles below. Here, the larger speech bubbles dominate the smaller speech bubbles. The smaller speech bubbles represent the person reflecting, while the larger ones represent the person guiding the reflection. In both examples, we can see the person guiding the reflection butting in, either turning the conversation towards themself or jumping in to offer advice. How might you respond if you were the person reflecting? I hope that over the next few pages you will be able to see this is *not* how reflective conversations should be experienced/facilitated and understand why.

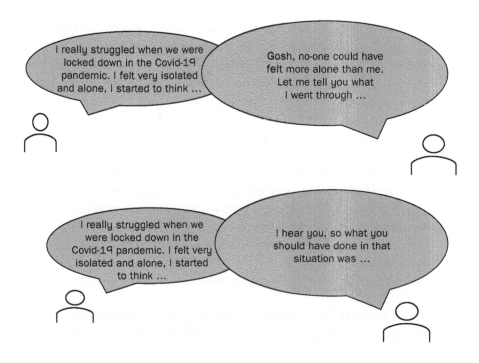

What is guided reflection?

Reflection empowers the reflector to have 'an authentic voice and one that enables them to talk about their experiences and their ability, or not, to learn from the work that they do' (Ghaye, 2000: 59). I want to remind us of what Ghaye brought to the forefront of our consciousness here. The notion of being the authentic self and empowering authenticity has been recognized as having significant importance for psychological wellbeing and personal growth since the inception of humanistic psychology and the work of central figures such as Carl Rogers and Abraham Maslow (Sanders, 2006). More recently, Boyraz and Kuhl (2015) found that people who engaged in reflection had higher levels of self-perceived authenticity, which led to increased life satisfaction and reduced distress. Clarke (2022) highlights the importance of providing time out for reflection to allow ourselves to honestly acknowledge and explore our thoughts and feelings. She advised that this is a self-caring and validating behaviour that allows for exploration of the authentic self. A guided reflective conversation should therefore enable exploration of the self and provide a space for you as the reflector to have an authentic voice, so that you are connecting with you. So, in essence,

> *Guided reflective conversation is a space for you as the reflector to reflect on your experiences with another person in a one-to-one situation or in a group setting (yes, we can also reflect in groups!). To be supported by another individual to be your authentic self and explore deeply the meaning of your experiences. Guided reflection is a space created between people with the purpose of empowering the person or persons reflecting to explore what constitutes 'I', in a manner that allows connection of the self to the experience. Guided reflection creates a space that facilitates discovery about the self, and the internal and external influencing factors on how the self was within the experience. Guided reflection will also support the reflector to compassionately challenge inherent assumptions and subjective bias that can inhibit the acquisition of knowledge that can lead to greater levels of self-awareness.*

The guided reflective conversation will require the facilitator to lead you into thinking deeply about your experiences; the facilitator, using specific communication skills and a specific attitude towards you and the conversation, will *push* you with respect and compassion, into thinking analytically and critically about your experiences and will facilitate your movement through the reflective process depicted in Chapters 1 and 7. As Dewey stated, 'While we cannot learn or be taught to think, we do have to learn how to think well, especially how to acquire the general habit of reflecting' (1933: 35). The person guiding you as reflector should support you in learning how to think well. What is important to note is this conversation can occur either formally or informally. A specific time and space can be created to purposefully explore an experience, or it can occur in more general conversation. The reflective conversation is very versatile. I have often guided my daughter to explore experiences she has had at school, or socially with her friends and part-time job. I have not meant for these conversations to be formally guided reflection; I am her mum after all – and sometimes mums just need to offer advice. But when I have recognized her need to be able to express herself, to have an authentic voice and to come to her own conclusions, I have borrowed skills and ways of being from the guided reflective conversation. I think that at times she has taken more from this than had I just jumped in and told her what to do, think or say!

Before we move on, I want to touch briefly upon *guided discovery*. What occurs within the reflective conversation is very similar to guided discovery, which is a concept usually associated with counselling practice. Guided discovery, and here you will see the similarities, is a conversation that uses open and exploratory questions to uncover information that is not immediately known to the person, which enables reflection to occur, and a synthesis of the information uncovered (Padesky and Greenberger, 1995). Furthermore, Neenan built on this by advising that a 'guided discovery approach would want to pursue ... personal meaning ... and is based on a genuine curiosity about where the questioning will lead, what might be uncovered and what the person will do with this material' (2009: 251). And Overholser (1993, 2018) suggests allowing for the development of new perspectives. So, guided discovery is not too dissimilar from guided reflective conversation, as the guided reflective conversation guides discovery of self with the purpose of generating meaning.

Exercise 9.2: Experiences of guided reflective conversations

How does what you now know compare to what you wrote down in the first exercise in this chapter?

Now, tell me about a time you experienced guided reflection. What was it like for you? How does it compare to the discussion we have just had? How did it leave you feeling? Did you learn anything about yourself?

What the reflective conversation is and is not!

We have now established a general understanding of what the guided reflective conversation is, so at this point I wish to explore further what it is and what it also is not. When you experience being guided through the reflective process, it is important to know what you should not be on the receiving end of. I wish for you to maintain a healthy, wonderful relationship with reflection. Should you experience poor or inappropriate guided reflection, this will frame your perspective of reflection in this way and could prevent further engagement with it – which, obviously, would be a shame.

Have a go at the following exercise.

Exercise 9.3: Experiences of conversations?

Think about all the different types of conversations you have had with many different people over the years. Using the framework below, jot down the positive things that helped to create a sense of feeling 'okay' within and after a conversation. Then, jot down those things that left you feeling somewhat uncomfortable. I don't want you to consider at this point what you did, but what the other person did. You do not need to name the person in your conversations or identify them. We are just listing general communication and attitudinal factors. I'll start you off with a couple of each from my own experiences.

Positive factors	*Negative factors*
Laughed at my jokes Smiled at me (smiled with their eyes)	Didn't even look up from their mobile phone Looked bored

Reflecting on your own experiences of conversations with others will help you to know what you want from a person who you allow to guide you in reflecting on your experiences. Let us now review what the reflective conversation is.

We can see from Figure 9.1 what the reflective conversation is and, coupled with our previous discussion, we should have a very clear understanding of what to expect from this type of conversation. But before we move on, I want to briefly touch upon 'owned by the reflector and can meander', as we have not previously discussed this.

What the reflective conversation is.

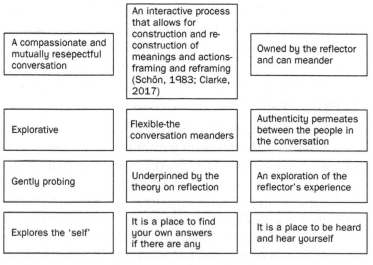

Figure 9.1 What the reflective conversation is

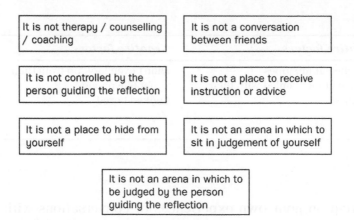

Figure 9.2 What the reflective conversation is not

The reflective conversation is not controlled by the facilitator, it is only controlled by the person reflecting (see Figure 9.2). The facilitator is there to support movement through the reflective process. But you as the person on the receiving end of guided reflection should feel in full control of the agenda and where you want the conversation to go. As the person being guided to reflect, you will need to mindfully connect with yourself, to allow your mind to take you wherever it wants to take you, even surprise you. I went to see 'Top Gun Maverick' twice at the cinema in one week. It was a very profound experience for me. So, I decided to reflect on it. I began by exploring my thoughts and feelings and investigating why I had responded to this film in the way I had, and before I realized I was recalling my youth and investigating the significance of zero responsibility, lost opportunities, and having an influence on my future decisions and happiness. This was highly unexpected, as my mind had meandered in a different direction, but to where it needed to go and meaningful nonetheless.

Your mind will carve out naturally what it wants you to discuss, and you will need to move with this by paying attention to yourself and going with your own flow. Johns (2002) used a zen poem that charted the aspects of a slow, fine stream that creates its own path between the obstacles that may get in its way, to eventually get to wherever it needs to go. I really liked the use of the metaphor of a stream to represent the fluidity of reflective dialogue. So, give yourself permission to go where you did not start out. This is the beauty of reflective dialogue as it should not be so structured that it becomes rigid. But it should be purposeful, yet just like the stream meandering along. Let us now look at what the reflective conversation is *not*.

What the reflective conversation is not

Take a look at figure 9.2. The reflective conversation is also not coaching. Coaching tends towards the use of quite specific models that are afforded acronyms that create a linear sequence that frames the coaching conversation. Such acronyms include RADAR – Rapport, Analyse, Demonstrate, Activity, Review (Giangregorio, 2016), previously and alternatively known as Relationship, Awareness, Dream, Action, Results/Review (Hilliard, 2012). One of the most used models in the UK is GROW – Goal, Reality, Options/Obstacles, Way forward (Tee et al., 2019). Tee and Passmore (2022) noted that coaching models can be overly relied upon by the practitioner and, by rigidly guiding the person they are helping through the model, the practitioner can gain a false sense of assurance they are acting as a practised and ethical coach and being useful. However, this overreliance on structure can inhibit the opportunity to maximize insight and learning from deep exploration and sense-making. The reflective conversation, on the other hand, engages in a process but does not adhere to a rigid linear structure. It is just as we have highlighted, a stream that meanders and flows through the process in whichever direction it does. The reflective models and frameworks discussed in the first edition of this book are not requirements for reflection and reflective practice to occur. Engagement in the reflective process is.

A reflective conversation is also not the same type of conversation you would have with your friends, where we will often compete to be heard, compare and contrast our stories, and offer each other advice. It is not a place where you will be judged on your thoughts, feelings and behaviours (the only caveat to this is if you are reflecting in a professional setting and your thoughts, feelings and behaviours pose a risk to others). It is not a place to hide from who you are, but to connect to yourself honestly and bravely.

In essence, therefore, the purpose of reflecting in a conversation is to:

- empower learning;
- support learning about self;
- enable/engender critical thinking;

- support the development of autonomous thinking;
- develop learning from experience;
- create a space for the facilitator to be a critical friend;
- create a framework for guided discovery to learn from experience

And you should perceive:

- that you are being listened to and heard;
- that a safe space has been created for conversation; and
- you are experiencing the facilitator as a sounding board – bouncing back your thoughts, supporting reframing of thinking, empowering development of new ways of perceiving.

Attitudinal qualities and skills required in the reflective conversation

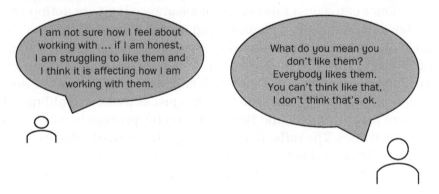

How might you feel if someone responded to you in the way shown above? I would like you to re-read what you wrote down for Exercise 9.3. Take another look at what you wrote about those conversations where you walked away feeling good about them. You may walk away from a reflective conversation feeling challenged, or feeling tired, or feeling excited, even rejuvenated – or you may walk away disappointed in the attitude you showed, or a behaviour you displayed towards something in your life. But you should *never* walk away feeling bad about yourself because of how you have been treated within the conversation by the person guiding the conversation.

Throughout the previous chapters in this book, we have explored the attitudinal qualities required to become an effective reflective practitioner. We are now going to explore how these relate to and underpin the reflective conversation. Before we focus on you as the reflector, let's explore the attitudinal qualities required of the facilitator so that you are choosy when it comes to who you allow to support your reflection.

Take a look at the list in Box 9.1. Are there any other qualities you would like to add? When we think about the above, we can see that qualities such as compassion, having respect for the process, being empathic, and where the person has a genuine wish to understand you from your own unique perspective, will not sit in judgement of you but values you, is open and honest about who they are – that is what creates that safe space for you to get to know you. A person who truly wants to hear what you have to say and has respect for the process of reflection as they model themselves what it is to be a reflective practitioner, is a person who has the attitudinal qualities to facilitate reflection in another.

Box 9.1: Qualities required of the facilitator

- Confidential – does not talk about you outside of the conversation
- Compassionate
- Confident
- Empathic
- Genuine / congruent
- Honest
- Reflective
- Respectful towards the process
- Respectful towards you
- Someone you have respect for
- Safe
- Self-aware
- Trustworthy
- Someone who shows unconditional positive regard
- Values you
- Someone who listens to you and hears you

In previous chapters, we explored what it is to be person-centred in the reflective process, discussed the core conditions of empathy and unconditional positive regard and their relationship to the reflective process. As we can see from Figure 9.3, these core conditions also have a role for the facilitator of reflection. Carl Rogers (1980), a prominent psychologist who we have met on several occasions already, authored many seminal works that laid down the theory underpinning what it is to be person-centred, and referred to the notion of person-centredness as a *way of being*. A *way of being* in the sense that the person embraces the conditions as principles and embodies the principles in every living moment rather than adopting them as specific professional practices at specific times. The qualities specified in Figure 9.3 need to be part of a *way of being* for the facilitator of reflection. Personally, I would not want to be guided in my reflections by an individual who only once in while is trustworthy, or who only adopts empathy when it suits them.

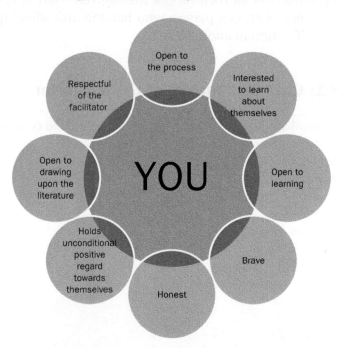

Figure 9.3 The attitudinal qualities required of the reflector

So, the attitudinal qualities of the person who you allow to facilitate your reflection is important. You will notice I keep referring to *who you allow*, since supporting a person to reflect is a privilege, not a right. So be mindful and choose a person who embodies what it is to be a reflective practitioner and sees it as *a way of being*.

Let us now remind ourselves of what attitudinal qualities you will need to receive guided reflection. Based upon what you know from having read the previous chapters, have a go at the following exercise.

Exercise 9.4: The reflector's attitudinal qualities

Jot down what attitudinal qualities you think you will need to receive guided reflection from another individual.

We previously discussed in detail the attitudinal qualities you will require as a reflector. Those same qualities are required when receiving guided reflection. Figure 9.3 reminds us of some of those qualities but with the added quality of being respectful of the facilitator. The reflective conversation is a two-way process: two people connect, two people are in a space together, two people are investigating experience. So, it is important to be considerate of the person guiding the reflection. But you also need to enter the process with an open mindset, a mindset for learning, being courageous, honest and kind to yourself.

Experiencing the reflective conversation

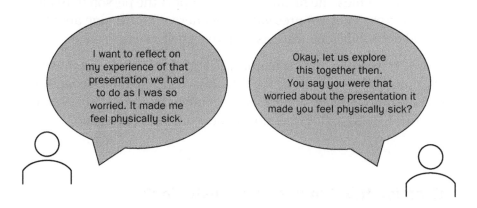

We know from our previous discussion that guiding discovery is not about changing minds or requiring the individual to come around to our way of thinking. The questioning style when guiding discovery is based on 'a genuine curiosity about where the questioning will lead, what might be uncovered and what the person will do with this material' (Neenan, 2009: 251). By looking at the speech bubbles above you should be able to see a clear difference in the facilitator's response to the individual reflecting compared with the responses in the speech bubbles earlier in the chapter. Here, you should be able to see a question is asked that, when coupled with the appropriate non-verbal communication, should convey a genuine curiosity on the part of the person guiding the reflection.

Genuine curiosity can also help make connections between experiences. Connelly and Clandinin suggested that 'narrative inquirers do not describe an event, person, or object as such, but rather describe them with a past, a present, and a future' (2006: 479). The authors termed this a temporal history. Greenberger et al. agreed with this and advised that reflective conversation will empower exploration of the reflector's narrative that is a 'three-dimensional expression of one's past, present, and future' (2021: 6). They further suggested that this temporal history helps the reflector to make connections between how the past affects the present, which will affect the future. Chapter 10 introduces us to Bassot's mirrors, and the importance of the rear view mirror in determining how what went before and is behind us will determine movement forward. It is hoped that you will experience your facilitator supporting you to make connections between past, present and future. In the subject matter of the conversation in the speech bubbles, the facilitator may support the person to explore previous experiences of presenting to generate knowledge about the past and determine connections with this current experience.

To help you to reflect, the facilitator will display several communication skills, one of which will be active listening. When nursing students are asked what communication skills are important, they almost always say active listening. But what do we mean by active listening?

Exercise 9.5: What is active listening?

Take a few minutes to think about your answer to this question. What would you write in your essay about active listening?

When you are being actively listened to, you will likely feel you have been heard and understood, that the reflector is only concerned with what you have experienced; that they are solely focused on observing you, hearing you and helping you to make connections; that they are picking up on your non-verbal cues, that you shouldn't feel hurried, and they want you to feel like sharing your story with them. The person who is actively listening will encourage you to respond to their verbal and non-verbal communication, prompting you to explore, leaning forward (but not in your space) to convey interest in you. They will look at you appropriately, they will not look bored or glaze over, and they won't be tempted to check the time or answer their phone. An active listener will remember words and phrases you have used and will help you to make connections to the words and phrases you use. Take a look at the speech bubbles below.

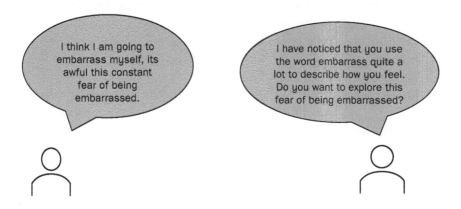

Driscoll (2000: 112) noted that people who do not actively listen will relate what they hear to themselves and will constantly interrupt and will 'need reminding of what has been said' by the reflector. So, you can see that this is an important skill for you as a facilitator of reflection to have. I remember paying for counselling many years ago and the counsellor kept looking out of the window and checking their watch. I was quite unhappy about this, and eventually got up and respectfully left.

We know from previous chapters that part of the reflective process is a critical and analytical exploration of experience. So, to help you go deeper into the analysis of your experience, the facilitator will use another communication skill, Socratic questioning. We have explored the idea of this form of questioning previously and it is this type of questioning that promotes self-discovery (Kidd, 1992) and serves 'to propel you forward, while your answers steer the direction of the dialogue' (Overholser, 2013: 74). This method of questioning is, of course, named after the Greek philosopher Socrates, and it focuses on asking a person a series of open-ended questions which can produce knowledge that is 'currently outside of their awareness and thereby enable the person to develop more helpful perspectives' (Neenan, 2009: 250). This method of probing one's experience should help you to reach your own conclusions and synthesize your own knowledge.

Read the following interaction between a reflector and facilitator:

> Reflector: *'I wasn't too sure about that lecture on harm reduction.'*
> Facilitator: *'Why not?'*
> Reflector: *'Well, I don't know ... it just felt uncomfortable.'*
> Facilitator: *'Why did it?'*
> Reflector: *'Mmm ... I'm not sure. It made me wonder whether I could adopt that approach.'*
> Facilitator: *'Why?'*
> Reflector: *'Well ...'*

A *why* question can be a Socratic question. But it can also be over-used. Overholser (2013) advised us that *why* questions are rarely helpful as people do not always know *why*. Imagine a child – children are amazing at asking *why?* But the more *why* questions they ask, the more the parent runs out of explanations. The above dialogue highlights the overuse of the *why* question and, when you read it, it reads like an inquisition, and I can guarantee that if you were the reflector here, it would feel like an inquisition. As a result, the person reflecting here shuts down. They don't know what more to say. This unhelpful line of Socratic questioning prompts closure rather than exploration, so the analysis is lost and exploration stops.

Now read the following piece of dialogue:

> Reflector: *'I think my mentor is amazing. She is such a good leader and so supportive.'*

Facilitator: *'It sounds like you have come away from placement having enjoyed your experience with your
mentor. You mentioned you think she is amazing,
did you feel supported by her?'*

Reflector: *'Absolutely. I was never anxious on placement
like I have been before.'*

Facilitator: *'So, this experience with her has been different to
your previous experiences which you say have
made you feel anxious. What do you think has
been different for you that you had not experienced before?'*

Reflector: *'Well, if I wasn't sure about anything she would
always take time to answer questions, I never felt
stupid. I have felt stupid for asking questions
before. She did not make me feel stupid.'*

Facilitator: *'She helped you to feel heard?'*

Reflector: *'Yes, she was like that with others too, not just me.
I think I actually did far more on this placement
than I have done previously.'*

Facilitator: *'Her supportive nature and feeling heard, do you
think this helped you in being able to do more,
maybe in developing your confidence to do more?'*

Reflector: *'I think so. I think I was less afraid of being told
off or embarrassed if I didn't do it right.'*

I guess you can see the difference in questioning here. It doesn't read
like an inquisition – it reads like the reflector is the focus of the conversation, that they are being heard and hopefully understood. The
questions at times and assumptions made on behalf of the facilitator
should be tentative and you should be empowered to correct their
understanding as in the above. The reflective conversation and the
Socratic questioning used should help you to clarify understanding,
challenge your assumptions, support evidence and reasoning for the
way you think, empower you to see your experience from alternative
viewpoints, help you to explore the implications and consequences of
your thinking/feeling/behaviours, and enable you to challenge questions you ask. This type of questioning, when applied appropriately
– and when combined with the skill of empathic responding – is what
can guide you into analytical exploration of your experience that will
generate knowledge about you (see Table 9.1).

Table 9.1 Socratic questioning

Clarification	What do you mean when you say X? Could you explain that point further? Can you provide an example?
Challenging assumptions	Is there a different point of view? What assumptions are we making here? Are you saying that …?
Evidence and reasoning	Can you provide an example that supports what you are saying? Can we validate that evidence? Do we have all the information we need?
Alternative viewpoints	Are there alternative viewpoints? How could someone else respond?
Implications and consequences	How would this affect someone? Are there any long-term implications of this?
Challenging the question	What do you think was important about that question? Was there a different question to ask?

In this chapter, we have explored what a reflective conversation is and is *not*. I hope you now have a good idea of what to expect when you allow a person to guide reflection in you. You should understand what to look for in a person *you allow* to support reflective conversation and guided discovery within you. I think we can safely say that the reflective conversation requires a particular attitude on behalf of both the reflector and facilitator and a significant skill set. This is no ordinary conversation. You may even want to have a go yourself. If you practise with another student, you will get a good feel for what works and what's not so good, which will allow you to gain more knowledge of reflective conversations whilst developing your own skill set.

Key points that can be taken from this chapter are:

- The reflective conversation is no ordinary conversation.
- Attitudinal qualities play an important role in the reflective conversation.
- A significant skill set is required on behalf of the facilitator of the reflective conversation.
- You allow an individual to facilitate reflection within you.
- The essence is on self-discovery.

Final thoughts and recommendations

In the first edition of the book, the equivalent to this chapter opened with the following quote.

> Two fundamental skills necessary for all healthcare profession-
> als are firstly, to discover and reflect on their own voice and
> secondly to enable others to hear and claim their own.
>
> (Ghaye, 2000: 55)

I decided to use it again as I still believe what Ghaye is saying here encapsulates the essence of the whole book. Finding your own authentic, reflective voice, validating your own narrative, lifting your head up long enough to explore the meaning of this narrative and how it influences every aspect of who you are, displaying a gen-uine curiosity about yourself, and then developing the skills to empower another person to do the same, is a skill set that you can use in every facet of your life – and in a positive way!

We have, throughout this book, discovered our voice: our reflective voice. I hope as a result you feel empowered to be the *best version of yourself*.

Learning outcomes

By the end of this chapter, you will be able to:

● Review and consolidate your knowledge of reflection and reflective practice.
● Review how the ten essential ingredients support movement
through the reflective process.
● Recognize potential barriers to reflection and explore strategies
to counteract them.
● Understand how different types of mirrors as metaphors for
reflection are useful in highlighting different angles through
which we can explore our experiences.
● Explore any gaps in our knowledge relating to this subject matter.

Let us recap briefly the fundamental purpose of reflection that we explored in Chapter 1. Take a look at Figure 10.1.

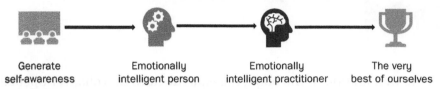

| Generate self-awareness | Emotionally intelligent person | Emotionally intelligent practitioner | The very best of ourselves |

Figure 10.1 The fundamental purpose of reflection

In Chapter 1, we explored in detail the notion of reflection. We came to know that the purpose of reflection is to empower us to be the *best version of ourselves*, not – as often thought – a 'better' version. For me, this is one of the most important takeaways from this book. Reflection is not about being a better you. The reflective process does not reduce you to a negative version of yourself and assume you must strive to be better, neither does it assume your professional practice in whatever field you work in requires improvement. Instead, it assumes that you would like to have more information and knowledge about yourself and how you are positioned within and influenced by your lived experiences. After all, knowledge is power and it is this power that will empower you to be the *best version of yourself*, in whatever guise that may be. The reflective process knows that our experiences contain information and, if we can unearth this information, we can create sense-making by generating the information to understand the context of ourselves.

If we review the revised extended description of reflection, we can see all that we have discussed encapsulated here (Box 10.1).

Box 10.1: A revised extended description of reflection

Reflection is an essential, engaging process that allows the reflector to frame and reframe their reality that is, and has been experienced moment by moment. Actively participating in the reflective process – that is, in, on or before an experience – requires us to tell our story and meander through that narrative, allowing ourselves to move where our thoughts and feelings wish to take us. It requires us to utilize skills of communication, to communicate with ourselves authentically, to become our own person-centred enquirer, understanding ourselves in relation to experiences we are about to have, are having or have had, empathically and with accuracy. Then stepping beyond the self and using this knowledge gained to understand how we may then have influenced those around us. To be fully immersed in this process, we must be open to learning about what constitutes 'I', leaving arrogance and complacency at the door, be kind and compassionate enough to offer ourselves unconditional positive regard, be actively engaged in mindfulness, and consciously aware of the self in our moments. Through a critical, analytical lens, we need to explore our experiences within the frame of how our history/background and current locus, culture and context influence who we are in our moments. Reflection requires us to open ourselves up to sourcing and learning new knowledge if the knowledge is not already known to us. And using that new knowledge gained to fill gaps in our current knowledge, challenge our preconceived notions and assumptions, and offer alternative ways of viewing experience to generate sense-making, thus creating information that can lead to personal and professional development. When we are fully open to and engaged in the process, reflection has the potential to empower us to be the best version of ourselves and inform our future experiences.

By viewing reflection as it is laid down here in this description, and throughout the chapters in this book, I hope you are now familiar with and comfortable with the notion of reflection, what it is and what its purpose is. We have secured an understanding of the process-orientated nature of reflection, of the learning that can occur within the process not just as a result of completing that process. We have developed our understanding of the significance of our narrative, the possibilities of storytelling and the power of journaling to support you in empowering your authentic voice.

We have a developed an understanding of how to explore our narrative to generate sense-making, to be able to formulate conclusions that contain knowledge that we can use to inform our future experiences in whatever manner we choose. We have constructed ways to enable us to view how we are influenced by our *provenance* (history/background), which in turn is influenced by our culture and the context of each experience we have. We have come to understand that we can be affected by those around us and in turn affect those others within our experiences. Our experiences do not occur in isolation – we do not *experience* in isolation. We affect others and in so doing generate knowledge of who we are. We have also come to know the significance of the external environment and its influence on how we think, feel and behave within our experiences.

Importantly, we now have two new reflective frameworks to work with, both of which emerged organically from the reflective process. We have **EESI** – **E**xperience, **E**xploration, **S**ense-making, **I**mplementation – a new reflective framework to support us mostly in reflecting on or pre-experience. And we have **EDI** – **E**xperience, **D**econstruction, **I**mplementation – to support writing reflectively for academic assessments. Both will help you to move fluidly through the reflective process. Also, in the previous chapter, we discussed in some detail facilitated reflection through conversation. All nurses, together with students in the health, education and life sciences professions, will take part in facilitated reflective discussion at some point, so it is important to be aware of what such a conversation entails.

Now, let us consider a question I also asked in the first edition of this book. Is there anything about the extended description of reflection you still don't understand? For example, is there anything you are unsure of or any elements that we have not covered, discussed or learned about in the previous chapters? If there are, jot these down and revisit the chapters in this book to try and uncover further knowledge to aid your understanding. You can also widen your reading as there are some wonderful writers on reflection out there to be discovered by you.

I hope that by reading this book you have grasped the notion that reflecting requires you to immerse yourself in the process of reflection. That there isn't a prescriptive means by which reflection can occur. That fundamentally being able to reflect requires theoretical knowledge of what it is, a skill set and a particular attitude towards the process. The revised extended description and our unique approach to reflection – the ten essential ingredients – offer us a new way of reflecting that considers the attitude and skills required and our own individuality by not prescribing *how to*. It communicates to the reflector what is needed for effective reflection and allows the reflector to review their attitude and skills in light of these requirements, while highlighting areas for development.

Let us look again at the ten essential ingredients for successful reflection and, unlike in Chapter 1, where we first met them, look at each of them alongside their unique narrative. These ingredients and their descriptions have been reviewed and modified in consideration of my own developmental reflective journey. The ingredients are addressed in the same order as they appeared in Chapters 2–6 (see Table 10.1).

Table 10.1 The ten essential ingredients for successful reflection

Critical analysis	Reflecting does not stop at the experience, but continues with an exploration of the experience prior to, during or after, through a critical, analytical lens. This critical analysis is inquisitive in nature, embodying curiosity and generated by the need to make sense of the experience and the quest for knowledge, particularly knowledge that can bridge the theory–practice gap and so be meaningful to the practice or personal experience. New knowledge gained is then amalgamated with the old and current knowledge, from which the person can then synthesize a new way of being leading to transformational change or expand and develop the current way of being.
Knowledge	The individual, in order to analyse, and reflect upon what they are experiencing in the clinical or personal setting, needs to have a level of knowledge that they can refer to and position their experience within. This knowledge enables objectivity to be brought into the subjective, filling knowledge gaps and challenging perception. If they do not have the existing knowledge, they need to know how to source the knowledge so that they may bridge that theory–practice gap and enhance their ability to understand the experience they are reflecting on.
Attitudinal qualities	The driving force of successful engagement with the reflective process. The individual needs to be humble to the process, be open, honest and willing, having the motivation to understand and learn about themselves. The individual needs to be brave, courageous and confident in order to encourage the honesty required in the process. Offering yourself kindness, compassion and unconditional positive regard enables openness and empowers the person reflecting to connect with their authentic self.

(continued)

Table 10.1 (Continued)

Self-awareness	The individual needs to have an existing level of awareness of self, a perception of how they recognize themselves to be. It is this current knowledge of self that is the basis for exploring the self within the reflective process. Self-awareness allows the individual to be honest about how they perceive themselves to be in the experience. It is this existing knowledge of the self that is also agreed, challenged, developed and overturned in, and by, the exploration that occurs within the reflective process – leading to new knowledge of self and potential transformational change.
Being person-centred	The person reflecting has vast resources for self-understanding. These resources for self-understanding can be accessed if we are person-centred with ourselves. Recognizing we have our own unique subjective view of the world (our individual phenomenology) allows us to create a climate whereby we can get to know ourselves and gain a deeper understanding of ourselves in relation to our experiences. With understanding, a heightened level of self-awareness grows. We are able to develop both personally and professionally.
Being empathic	The person reflecting needs to want to understand themselves in relation to their experiences accurately. They need to use the skills of empathic questioning and responding to allow for deeper analysis and as a result understanding and sense-making of their thoughts, feelings and behaviour in relation to the experience they are reflecting on. Not only this, they need also to be able to use their empathy to understand how others perceive them and the experience they have been part of.
Communication	The person reflecting needs to be able to articulate in a verbal and non-verbal manner, whether this is to themselves or to another person. They need to have the communication skills that allow them to act as their own internal supervisor. These communication skills include the skills of Socratic questioning and empathic responding in order to be able to investigate and enquire deeply into their experiences.
Mindfulness	The person reflecting needs to be present with themselves, aware of how their surroundings are and will guide their behaviours, thoughts and feelings within experiences. An acute awareness of how their values and belief systems, along with culture, policy and the political sphere will influence who they are in the context of others.

(continued)

Table 10.1 (Continued)

Being process-orientated	Reflection is not about the outcome/output, but about the process that takes place when reflecting. Reflection may not always be so smooth as to guarantee a definitive outcome. When entering the reflective process, the person reflecting needs to meander and follow their own flow of feeling or train of thought. As much learning can take place from the process as can occur from the result.
Being deliberate	Reflecting is not a flippant, inconsequential recap of an event, but a deliberate, controlled, conscious, exploratory consideration of an experience. It is not just thinking! Engaging in the reflective process gives the reflector permission to take purposeful time to stop and spend moments with themselves. The reflector must also be cognisant that every decision they make as a result of reflection has a 'ripple effect'. The actions they take from the reflective process will not only impact upon the person reflecting but on those around them.

Here we have our unique approach to successful reflection, the ten essential ingredients; ingredients that establish the need for the person reflecting to want to get to know who they are and adopt a certain attitude and way of thinking about themselves. To hold a certain mentality towards the reflective process, to position themselves within the person-centred paradigm within which they can safely and comfortably analyse and explore their experiences, getting to know their genuine self. This approach, underpinned by the ten essential ingredients, requires the reflector to recognize the need to harness the intellectual, academic skills not always associated with reflection, using the knowledge we already have to position and frame our experience and identify those areas where further research is required. Ingredients that empower the reflector to understand the value in the process, to recognize the learning that also takes place as we reflect. At the end of each chapter where these ingredients are located and explored, the relevant part of the revised extended description provides a visual connection between the ingredients and the description itself.

As I stated in the first edition of the book, using these ingredients for reflection is akin to mixing the ingredients to bake a cake. The blending together and baking of these ingredients gives us the final product – a successful reflective practitioner.

Before we move on, I would like us to touch upon something we have not yet discussed, barriers to reflection. Now that you have significant knowledge of reflection, have a go at the following exercise.

Exercise 10.1: Barriers to reflection

After a few moments of reflection, jot down what you consider to be barriers to successful reflection. Then jot down what you think might be put in place to overcome these barriers. I'll start you off with one example.

Barriers/obstacles	*Enablers/assisters*
Lack of skills to facilitate reflection	Attend a course/training/research/ practice

Knowing that there are potential barriers to reflection is important. Being able to identify personal barriers, professional barriers and organizational barriers will enable you to be proactive in counteracting them. It may be that certain barriers will influence how you reflect and what you reflect about. A personal barrier, for example, might be you not being ready to fully reflect on an experience – that your mind is not present enough with the experience to analyse and explore. So, your enabler might be to journal and connect with yourself enough to help tell your important authentic story, until you are ready to explore. Knowing and understanding barriers to reflection can act as an enabler.

Mirrors as a metaphor for reflection

Before we conclude our final chapter, I want to introduce you to Bassot's (2020) metaphorical mirrors. Using different types of mirrors as metaphors, Bassot was able to demonstrate the different angles, views or perspectives reflection can give us about our experiences. I have personally found these mirrors extremely helpful when teaching my students the usefulness of reflection and how it can really focus in on and highlight different sides to our experiences. So let us take a brief look at these mirrors (Bassot, 2020: 6–7).

> **The bathroom mirror:** This mirror reflects in the traditional sense exactly how other people view us. Bassot's (2020) interpretation of this mirror is that we can accept how the world sees us, or we can make a conscious decision to make ourselves more presentable.

I do not agree that this mirror helps us to decide if we need to look more presentable to the outside world because, yet again, we are reducing ourselves to something less than and judging ourselves as not being good enough. However, the immediacy of this mirror allows us to determine if this is how we wish to represent ourselves to the outside world. When I am teaching and I look at myself in that morning bathroom mirror, I want to present myself to my students as a person that perceives what I do as important, that being with them in a learning moment is important to me, so I make an effort with how I present myself. I clean my teeth, brush my hair, and so on. The message conveyed from the morning bathroom mirror is 'I have just got up' – this is not the message I wish to convey to my students!

The immediacy of how I came across to the outside world was evident in a moment when I was a student. In a moment when undertaking group work, a peer held up that bathroom mirror and reflected back to me that I was a *bossy cow*! This was like a punch to the gut. But I took it on the chin as this was how I was presenting to the outside world, and explored this, as this was not how I wanted to be perceived by others. I did not wish to lose my assertiveness, but I did not wish either to be perceived by others as being bossy.

> **The rear view mirror:** This mirror represents the car rear view mirror, and Bassot (2020) reminds us of the importance of the information this mirror contains about how our past will inform how we move forward in our future.

I often ask my students, 'Who drives a car? And if you do, how often do you use your rear view mirror?' We laugh together as we discuss how the rear view mirror shows a Range Rover hurtling up behind us, and which allows us to assess and analyse if we can safely overtake the car in front, in our Skoda Yeti. You'd be surprised how many people admit to not using their rear view mirror. Reflection via the rear view mirror – or on-experience as we might also call it – helps us to determine how our past self and past experiences can influence our future. It provides us with knowledge in every way we have discussed throughout this book.

Wing mirrors: Wing mirrors, according to Bassot (2020), give us the ability not only to view what is behind us but also the blind spots.

This mirror, different to the rear view mirror, highlights our blind spots. Blind spots in relation to our experiences are the aspects of the experience we perhaps cannot see, or the influence we do not know we have. When reflecting, we employ strategies to understand how we influence others. One example is to use Brookfield's (2017) Four Lenses of Critical Reflection to try and gain other people's perspectives on us, but we can also ask for feedback or, especially in professional practice, ask to be observed. These are ways in which we can access our blind spots.

The magnifying mirror: Bassot states that the magnifying mirror 'is indispensable in situations where we need to look at our faces closely …'

(2020: 6).

Recognizing reflection as a mirror that can magnify will help you to focus in on the minutiae of an experience. You might find yourself returning over and over again to a particular aspect of an experience. If you do, then get out the reflection magnifying mirror and home in on that particular aspect. Use this mirror to blow it up, to make it bigger so you can start to understand how this one part connects to the whole experience and why it is your mind keeps wanting to take you back to it.

The funfair mirrors: These mirrors represent our ability to distort the narrative of our experience

(Bassot, 2020).

Thinking of looking into funfair mirrors when reflecting allows us to explore whether or not we have distorted our narrative, our story of the experience. We may have distorted it for a particular reason that is as yet not known to us. We may need to feel guilty because, paradoxically, feeling guilty can help us to feel better about something. When I was a student nurse on my very first mental health placement, I went and said good morning to a patient and asked them how they were. The patient yelled at me very loudly, *'how did I think they were, what a stupid question to ask'*. I ran out of the day room and spent the rest of the evening telling myself I was an awful student, I would make a terrible mental health nurse and that I had probably made this patient ill! From this experience I internalized that patient's entire issues as being my fault. Of course, it wasn't my fault, I had only met them that day. But I distorted my narrative. I didn't like being away from home, I wasn't sure I wanted to do nursing, I had distorted to give myself an excuse to drop out of my course! – I didn't drop out though because the next day a wonderful mentor helped me to reflect and empowered me to normalize my distorted image. I then had to reflect on why I had thought I didn't want to be a nurse.

> **Shop windows:** Although these are not true mirrors, 'we can see our reflection [in them] as we walk past'. Bassot sees them as a way of 'think[ing] about things as we are doing something else'
> (2020: 7).

Bassot (2020) likens this to reflecting in-experience or in-action. Whilst we are doing something we might consider in the moment how to do it differently, or consider how the person we are doing something with is responding to us, or how we are responding to them. We might continue *doing*, whilst thinking all this through and considering other ways of doing, being, behaving and so on.

So we can see that Bassot uses mirrors to help us to acknowledge all the different ways in which we can view our experiences and use reflection to do so. I find the rear view and wing mirror metaphors particularly useful in helping me to recognize how my past can influence my future, and how important being able to see my blind spots is in relation to enabling me to be the *best version of myself*. Which one resonates most with you?

Let us now consolidate everything that we have learned by reading this book. Have a go at the following exercise.

Exercise 10.2: Consolidating knowledge

We now know what reflection is and we have our revised extended description. We also have the ten essential ingredients that make up the reflective process and we understand that the key to adult, transformational learning is the reflective conversation we have with ourselves or another person or persons. With that in mind, have a go at answering the following questions:

- What do you now understand reflection to be?
- Do you think the ten essential ingredients are a necessary part of reflection?
- How would you use the ten essential ingredients?
- Which chapter of the book did you find the most useful and why?
- When do you think you will find reflection most helpful?
- How do you feel about reflection now?
- How might you share what you now know with others?

Finally, here are my recommendations based upon many years of engaging with reflection. Please feel free to add to or modify this list to suit your own needs.

Recommendations for successful reflection

- Accept reflection as needing to be a natural part of who you are.
- Embody what it is to be a successful reflective practitioner/person.
- As well as reflecting on professional experiences, reflect also on experiences outside your professional practice.
- Telling your narrative/story is where authenticity occurs and is the most important aspect of the reflective process.
- Ensure you reflect through that critical analytical lens.
- Journaling is powerful.

- Literature, theory and evidence have an important role to play in the reflective process, bringing some objectivity into the subjective, offering new perspectives and filling gaps in your knowledge.
- Practise reflecting as often as you can.
- Reflect in a manner that suits you – remember, it can be messy and meandering.
- Ask your clinical mentors/personal tutors to offer you guided reflection. But be mindful of who you allow to guide you in the reflective conversation.
- Don't just reflect on the negative experiences you have.
- Recognize the value in reflecting on all types of experience you have.
- Initiate a reflective practice group with your peers where you can reflect together.
- Keep revisiting the revised extended description of reflection to ensure you understand the point of what we are doing here.
- View reflection as process-orientated and acknowledge the learning that takes place as part of this process.
- Remember to combine the ten essential ingredients when reflecting, in whatever mode and manner you reflect.
- Remember also to put into practice the learning that occurs as a result of reflecting.
- Reflection is *not* about being a better person or improving behaviours.

A final word

I wish to recall what I said in Chapters 1 and 10:

> 'I/you/we are the vessel through which the professional practice radiates. Moving beyond technical rationality and engaging in reflection, by delving into and exploring the messiness of the swampy lowlands – lowlands that contain the humanness of values, beliefs, feelings, interpersonal connections and the influence of culture, policy and politics – will allow you to be the master of your own vessel. The vessel which is the vehicle through which our practice emanates. Understanding your vehicle, learning to drive the vehicle of self with knowledge and authority, is what will enable you to be an amazing practitioner/professional. The reflective process knows that our experiences contain information and, if we can unearth this information, we can create sense-making by generating the information to understand the context of ourselves.'

As I said in the first edition of this book, practice makes perfect. By practising and perfecting the art of reflection and reflective practice, reflection will become a natural part of your everyday practice, and as a result not only will you become a more emotionally intelligent individual and practitioner, but you will become the *best version of yourself* in the different facets of your life. You will be capable of understanding yourself and how to use that understanding within the therapeutic relationships you have with those you care for, and in the relationships that shape your personal lives. You will understand the impact you have on others and be able to use that understanding to empathically *be* with another person.

I truly hope that you have enjoyed reading this second edition and taken some new insights from it that are helpful to understanding who you are.

References

Agnew, T. (2022) Reflective practice 1: aims, principles and role in revalidation, *Nursing Times*, 118: 5 [https://www.nursingtimes.net/clinical-archive/wellbeing-for-nurses/reflective-practice-1-aims-principles-and-role-in-revalidation-11-04-2022/].

Allport, G.W. (1935) Attitudes, in C. Murchison (ed.) *Handbook of Social Psychology*. Worcester, MA: Clark University Press.

Archer, M.S. (2007) *Making Our Own Way through the World: Human reflexivity and social mobility*. Cambridge: Cambridge University Press.

Atkins, S. (2004) Developing underlying skills in the move towards reflective practice, in C. Bulman and S. Schutz (eds.) *Reflective Practice in Nursing*, 3rd edition. Oxford: Blackwell.

Atkins, S. and Murphy, K. (1993) Reflection: a review of the literature, *Journal of Advanced Nursing*, 18 (8): 1188–92 [https://doi.org/10.1046/j.1365-2648.1993.18081188.x].

Bager-Charleson, S. (2010) *Reflective Practice in Counselling and Psychotherapy*. London: Sage.

Bandman, E.L. and Bandman, B. (1995) *Critical Thinking in Nursing*, 2nd edition. Norwalk, CT: Appleton & Lange.

Bassot, B. (2020) *The Reflective Journal*, 3rd edition. London: Bloomsbury.

Bolton, G. (2010) *Reflective Practice, Writing and Professional Development*, 3rd edition. London: Sage.

Bolton, G. and Delderfield, R. (2018) *Reflective Practice: Writing and professional development*. London: Sage.

Bond, M. and Holland, S. (1998) *Skills of Clinical Supervision for Nurses*. Buckingham: Open University Press.

Borton, T. (1970) *Reach, Touch and Teach*. London: Hutchinson.

Boyd, E. and Fales, A. (1983) Reflective learning: the key to learning from experience, *Journal of Humanistic Psychology*, 23 (2): 99–117 [https://doi.org/10.1177/0022167883232011].

Boyraz, G. and Kuhl, M.L. (2015) Self-focused attention, authenticity, and well-being, *Personality and Individual Differences*, 87: 70–75 [https://doi.org/10.1016/j.paid.2015.07.029].

Bozarth, J.D. (2002) Empirically supported treatment: epitome of the 'specificity myth', in J.C. Watson, R.N. Goldman and M.S. Warner (eds.) *Client-Centered and Experiential Psychotherapy in the 21st Century: Advances in theory, research, and practice*. Ross-on-Wye: PCCS Books.

Braillon, A. & Taiebi, F. (2020) Practicing "Reflective listening" is a mandatory prerequisite for empathy. *Patient Education and Counselling*, 103 (9): 1866–1867

Brammer, L.M. and MacDonald, G. (1996) *The Helping Relationship: Process and skills*, 6th edition. London: Allyn & Bacon.

Brockbank, A. and McGill, I. (2006) *Facilitating Reflective Learning through Mentoring and Coaching*. London: Kogan Page.

Brookfield, S. (2017) *Becoming a Critically Reflective Teacher*. San Francisco, CA: Jossey-Bass.

Butterworth, T., Carson, J., White, E. et al. (1997) It is Good to talk: An evaluation of clinical supervision and mentorship in England and Scotland. University of Manchester, Manchester.

Casement, P. (1985) *On Learning from the Patient*. New York: Guilford Press.

Chatfield, T. (2018) *Critical Thinking: Your guide to effective argument, successful analysis & independent study*. London: Sage.

Ciarrochi, J.V. and Bailey, A. (2008) *A CBT Practitioner's Guide to ACT: How to bridge the gap between cognitive behavioral therapy & acceptance & commitment therapy*. Oakland, CA: New Harbinger Publications.

Clarke, N.M. (2014) A person-centred enquiry into the teaching and learning experiences of reflection and reflective practice – part one, *Nurse Education Today*, 34 (9): 1219–24 [https://doi.org/10.1016/j.nedt.2014.05.017].

Clarke, N.M. (2017) *The Student Nurse's Guide to Successful Reflection: The ten essential ingredients.* London: Open University Press.

Clarke, N.M. (2021) Experience, Deconstruction, Implementation: EDI; a new approach to reflective writing for academic purpose, *Journal of Reflective Practice*, 22 (5): 714–26 [https://doi.org/10.1080/14623943.2021.1946775].

Clarke, N.M. (2022) Reflection is an often-misunderstood term, *Nursing Times*, 118: 5 [https://www.nursingtimes.net/opinion/reflection-is-an-often-misunderstood-term-within-nursing-13-04-2022/].

Connelly, F.M. and Clandinin, D.J. (2006) Narrative inquiry, in J. Green, G. Camilli and P. Elmore (eds.) *Handbook of Complementary Methods in Education Research*, 3rd edition. Mahwah, NJ: Lawrence Erlbaum Associates.

Dalley, J. (2009) Purpose and value in reflection, in H. Bulpitt and M. Deane (eds.) *Connecting Reflective Learning, Teaching and Assessment.* London: Higher Education Academy.

DaSilveira, A., DeSouza, M. L. and Gomes, W. B. (2015) Self-consciousness concept and assessment in self-report measures. *Frontiers in psychology*, 6: 930

Dewey, J. (1910) *How We Think.* New York: D.C. Heath.

Dewey, J. (1933) *How We Think: A restatement of the relation of reflective thinking to the educative process.* Boston, MA: D.C. Heath.

Dewing, J., McCormack, B. and McCance, T. (2021) *Person-Centred Nursing Research: Methodology, methods and outcomes.* Cham: Springer.

Dexter, G. and Wash, M. (2001) *Psychiatric Nursing Skills.* London: Thomas Nelson.

Diener, I., Kargela, M. & Louw, A. (2016) Listening is therapy: Patient interviewing from a pain science perspective. *Physiotherapy Theory and Practice*, 32 (5): 356–367

Driscoll, J. (2000) *Practising Clinical Supervision: A reflective approach.* London: Baillière Tindall.

Eagly, A.H. and Chaiken, S. (1998) Attitude structure and function, in D.T. Gilbert, S.T. Fiske and G. Lindzey (eds.) *The Handbook of Social Psychology*, 4th edition. New York: McGraw-Hill.

Eckroth-Bucher, M. (2010) Self-awareness: a review and analysis of a basic nursing concept, *Advances in Nursing Science*, 33 (4): 297–309 [https://doi.org/10.1097/ANS.0b013e3181fb2e4c].

Egege, S. (2020) *Becoming a Critical Thinker*. London: Macmillan Education.

Elliott, R., Bohart, A.C., Watson, J.C. and Greenburg, L.S. (2011) Empathy. *Psychotherapy*, 48 (1): 43–49

Ennis, R. (1996) Critical thinking dispositions: their nature and accessibility, *Informal Logic*, 18 (2/3): 165–82 [https://doi.org/10.22329/il.v18i2.2378].

Farrell, T. (2008) Reflective Language Teaching; *From Research to Practice*, pp. 1–4. London: Continuum Press.

Ghaye, T. (2000) The role of reflection in nurturing creative clinical conversations, in T. Ghaye and S. Lillyman (eds.) *Effective Clinical Supervision: The role of reflection*. Dinton, Wiltshire: Mark Allen.

Giangregorio, E. (2016) RADAR instructional coaching model, in D. Tee and J. Passmore (eds.) *Coaching Practiced*. Chichester: Wiley.

Gibbs, G. (1998) *Learning by Doing: A guide to teaching and learning methods*. Oxford: Further Education Unit.

Goleman, D. (2004) What Makes a Leader? *Harvard Business Review*, 82 (1): 82–91.

Greenberger, S.W., Maguire, K.R., Martin, C.L., et al. (2021) Discovering reflective-narrative: constructing experience in the Deweyan guide for reflective practice, *Reflective Practice*, 23 (2): 147–61 [https://doi.org/10.1080/14623943.2021.1983423].

Haley, B., Heo, S., Wright, P. et al. (2017) Relationships among active listening, self-awareness, empathy, and patient-centered care in associate and baccalaureate degree nursing students. *Nursing-Plus Open*, 3, pp.11–16.

Hanscomb, S. (2017) *Critical Thinking: The basics*. London: Routledge.

Health & Care Professions Council (HCPC) (2023) *Standards of Proficiency*. London: HCPC [https://www.hcpc-uk.org/standards/standards-of-proficiency/].

Hilliard, P. (2012) *Coaching Model: The RADAR*. International Coach Academy. Available at: https://coachcampus.com/coach-portfolios/coaching-models/pearl-hilliard-the-radar (accessed 15 May 2023).

Hofstadter, D. (2007) *I Am a Strange Loop*. New York: Basic Books.

Hogg, M. and Vaughan, G. (2005) *Social Psychology*, 4th edition. London: Prentice-Hall.

Jasper, M. (2013) *Beginning Reflective Practice*, 2nd edition. Andover: Cengage Learning.

Johns, C. (2000) *Becoming a Reflective Practitioner*. Oxford: Blackwell.

Johns, C. (2005) Expanding the gates of perception, in C. Johns and D. Freshwater (eds.) *Transforming Nursing Through Reflective Practice*, 2nd edition. Oxford: Blackwell.

Johns, C. (2010) *Guided Reflection: A narrative approach to advancing professional practice*. Chichester: Wiley.

Johns, C. (2022) *Becoming a Reflective Practitioner*. Hoboken, NJ: Wiley-Blackwell.

Kidd, I. (1992) *Socratic Questions*. New York: Routledge.

Kirschenbaum, H. and Henderson, V.L., eds. (1989) *The Carl Rogers Reader*. London: Constable.

Kirk, T.W. 2007 *Beyond empathy: clinical intimacy in nursing practice*, England.

Luft, J. and Ingham, H. (1955) *The Johari Window: A graphic model for interpersonal relations*. Los Angeles, CA: University of California Western Training Lab.

May, L. (2003) Support Systems. *Nursing Standard*, 17 (24): 60–62

McCormack, B. and McCance, T.V. (2006) Development of a framework for person-centred nursing, *Journal of Advanced Nursing*, 56 (5): 472–79 [https://doi.org/10.1111/j.1365-2648.2006.04042.x].

McCormack, B. and McCance, T. (2010) *Person-centred Nursing: Theory and practice.* Oxford: Wiley-Blackwell.

Mearns, D. and Thorne, B. (1988) *Person-centred Counselling in Action.* London: Sage.

Miller, W.R and Rollnick, S. (2002) *Motivational Interviewing: Preparing people for change.* New York: Guilford Press.

Milne, A. A. (1928) *The House at Pooh Corner.* London: Methuen.

Morse, J., Bottorff, J., Anderson, G. et al (1992) Beyond Empathy: Expanding expressions of caring. *Journal of Advanced Nursing.* 17: 809–821.

Myers, K.K., Krepper, R., Nilbert, A. & Toms, R. (2020) Nurses' Active Empathetic Listening Behaviours from the Voice of the Patient. *Nursing Economics,* 38 (5): 267–275

Neenan, M. (2009) Using Socratic questioning in coaching, *Journal of Rational-Emotive Cognitive-Behavior Therapy,* 27: 249–64 [https://doi.org/10.1007/s10942-007-0076-z].

Nelson-Jones, R. (2006) *Theory and Practice of Counselling and Therapy.* London: Sage.

Nursing and Midwifery Council (NMC) (2018a) *Future Nurse: Standards of proficiency for registered nurses.* London: NMC [https://www.nmc.org.uk/globalassets/sitedocuments/standards-of-proficiency/nurses/future-nurse-proficiencies.pdf].

Nursing and Midwifery Council (NMC) (2018b) *The Code: Professional standards of practice and behaviour for nurses, midwives and nursing associates.* London: NMC [https://www.nmc.org.uk/standards/code/].

Nursing and Midwifery Council (NMC) (2019) *Benefits of Becoming a Reflective Practitioner: A joint statement of support from Chief Executives of statutory regulators of health and care professionals.* London: NMC [https://www.nmc.org.uk/globalassets/sitedocuments/other-publications/benefits-of-becoming-a-reflective-practitioner---joint-statement-2019.pdf].

Overholser, J.C. (1993) Elements of the Socratic method: I. Systematic questioning, *Psychotherapy: Theory, Research, Practice, Training,* 30 (1): 67–74 [https://doi.org/10.1037/0033-3204.30.1.67].

Overholser, J.C. (2013) Guided discovery, *Journal of Contemporary Psychotherapy*, 43 (2): 73–82 [https://doi.org/10.1007/s10879-012-9229-1].

Overholser, J. (2018) *The Socratic Method of Psychotherapy*. New York: Columbia University Press.

Padesky, C.A. and Greenberger, D. (1995) *Clinician's Guide to Mind Over Mood*. New York: Guilford Press.

Paul, R. (1993) *Critical Thinking: What every person needs to survive in a rapidly changing world*. Santa Rosa, CA: Foundation for Critical Thinking.

Pinto, R.Z., Ferreira, M.L., Oliviera, V.C. et al (2012) Patient-centred communication is associated with positive therapeutic alliance: a systematic review. *Journal of Physiotherapy*, 58 (2): 77–87

Roberts, M. (2015) *Critical Thinking and Reflection for Mental Health Nursing Students*. London: Sage.

Robins, A., Ashbaker, B., Enriquez, J. and Morgan, J. (2003) Learning to reflect: professional practice for professionals and paraprofessionals, *International Journal of Learning*, 10: 2555–65.

Roche, J. and Harmon, D. (2017) Exploring the Facets of Empathy and Pain in Clinical Practice: A Review. *Pain Practice*, 17 (8): 1089–1096

Rogers, C.R. (1951) *Client-Centered Therapy*. Boston, MA: Houghton Mifflin.

Rogers, C.R. (1957) The necessary and sufficient conditions of therapeutic personality change, *Journal of Consulting Psychology*, 21 (2): 95–103 [https://doi.org/10.1037/h0045357].

Rogers, C.R. (1959) A theory of therapy, personality, and interpersonal relationships, as developed in the client-centered framework, in S. Koch (ed.) *Psychology: A study of a science, Vol. 3: Formulations of the person and the social context*. New York: McGraw-Hill.

Rogers, C.R. (1967) The interpersonal relationship in the facilitation of learning, in R. Leeper (ed.) *Humanizing Education*. Alexandria, VA: Association for Supervision and Curriculum Development.

Rogers, C.R. (1980) *A Way of Being*. Boston, MA: Houghton Mifflin.

Ryum, T., Stiles, T. C., Svartberg, M., & McCullough, L. (2010). The role of transference work: The therapeutic alliance and their interaction in reducing interpersonal problems among psychotherapy patients with cluster C personality disorders. *Psychotherapy: Theory, Research, Practice, Training*, 47: 442–453. doi:10.1037/a0021183

Sanders, P. (2006) *The Person-Centred Counselling Primer: A concise, accessible, comprehensive introduction*. Hereford: PCCS Books.

Schön, D.A. (1983) *The Reflective Practitioner: How practitioners think in action*. New York: Basic Books.

Smith, E. (2011) Teaching critical reflection, *Teaching in Higher Education*, 16 (2): 211–23 [https://doi.org/10.1080/13562517.2010.515022].

Taylor, B. (2000) *Reflective Practice: A guide for nurses and midwives*. Maidenhead: Open University Press.

Taylor, B. (2006) *Reflective Practice: A guide for nurses and midwives*, 2nd edition. Maidenhead: Open University Press.

Tee, D. and Passmore, J., eds. (2022) *Coaching Practiced*. Chichester: Wiley.

Tee, D., Passmore, J. and Brown, H. (2019) Distinctions in coaching practice between England and the rest of Europe, *The Coaching Psychologist*, 15 (2): 30–37.

Thompson, S. and Thompson, N. (2008) *The Critically Reflective Practitioner*. Palgrave: Macmillan.

Thompson, S. and Thompson, N. (2023) *The Critically Reflective Practitioner*. London: Bloomsbury.

Tobin, R. (2019) How objective and subjective storylines can improve your screenplay, *Creative Screen Writing*, 17 October https://www.creativescreenwriting.com/how-objective-and-subjective-storylines-can-improve-your-screenplay/.

Todd, G. (2002) The role of the internal supervisor in developing therapeutic nursing, in D. Freshwater (ed.) *Therapeutic Nursing: Improving patient care through self-awareness and reflection*. London: Sage.

Todd, G. (2005) Reflective practice and Socratic dialogue, in T. Ghaye and S. Lillyman (eds.) *Effective Clinical Supervision: The role of reflection*. Dinton, Wiltshire: Mark Allen.

Van Hooft, S., Gillam, L. and Byrnes, M. (1995) *Facts and Values: An introduction to critical thinking for nurses*. Sydney, NSW: MacLennan & Petty.

Van Manen, M. (1995) On the epistemology of reflective practice, *Teachers and Teaching: Theory and Practice*, 1 (1): 33–50 [https://doi.org/10.1080/1354060950010104].

Walsh-Burke, K. (2006) Grief and Loss: *Theories and Skills for Helping Professionals*, 1st edition. Boston: Pearson.

Wells, A. (1997) Cognitive therapy for anxiety disorder, in C. Johns and D. Freshwater (eds.) *Transforming Nursing Through Reflective Practice*, 2nd edition. Oxford: Blackwell.

White, D. (2004) Reflective practice: wishful thinking or a practical leadership tool?, *Practising Administrator*, 26 (3): 41–44.

Wieringa, N. (2011) Teachers' educational design as a process of reflection-in-action: the lessons we can learn from Donald Schon's The Reflective Practitioner when studying the professional practice of teachers as educational designers, *Curriculum Inquiry*, 41 (1): 167–74 [https://doi.org/10.1111/j.1467-873X.2010.00533.x].

Wilkinson, J.M. (1996) *Nursing Process: A critical thinking approach*. Reading, MA: Addison-Wesley.

Williams, K., Woolliams, M. and Spiro, J. (2012) *Reflective Writing*. Basingstoke: Palgrave Macmillan.

Winter, R. (1988) Fictional critical writing, in J. Nias and S. Groundwater-Smith (eds) *The Enquiring Teacher*. London: Routledge.

Wispé, L. (1986) The distinction between sympathy and empathy: a word is needed, *Journal of Personality and Social Psychology*, 50 (2): 314–21.

Index